THE EVERYTHING

DIABETES
COOKBOOK
2ND EDITION

Dear Reader,

Whether you have been newly diagnosed with diabetes or are someone who's had diabetes for a long time, you already understand that healthy eating and lifestyle changes are necessary components of diabetes management. This book is a resource designed to help you transition to a healthier way of eating and preparing food.

As a dietitian in private practice, I've had many new clients arrive at my office with the anticipation of being told their favorite foods are going to be taken away. After we discuss healthy eating strategies and review possible food options, most of my clients leave our initial meeting feeling pleasantly surprised. They have learned that a diabetic eating plan is about common sense and moderation, not deprivation.

This book has a wide array of recipes, some similar to your old favorites and some that are completely new and different. I would encourage you to try some new recipe ideas to expand your choices and add more variety to your food plan. You may also want to take the ideas suggested in this book and apply them to your own favorite recipes. Having diabetes does not mean you need to make separate meals or foods; the recipes and cooking methods described in this cookbook provide healthy options for everyone in your household.

Developing and testing the recipes I have included in this cookbook has been an enjoyable extension of my work as a Certified Diabetes Educator. When recipes result in great-tasting foods, cooking becomes a pleasure. It is my sincere hope that you enjoy using this cookbook and the recipes. I hope you will come away feeling pleasantly surprised!

Gretchen Scalpi, RD, CDN, CDE

Welcome to the EVERYTHING® Series!

These handy, accessible books give you all you need to tackle a difficult project, gain a new hobby, comprehend a fascinating topic, prepare for an exam, or even brush up on something you learned back in school but have since forgotten.

You can choose to read an *Everything*® book from cover to cover or just pick out the information you want from our four useful boxes: e-questions, e-facts, e-alerts, and e-ssentials.

We give you everything you need to know on the subject, but throw in a lot of fun stuff along the way, too.

We now have more than 400 *Everything*® books in print, spanning such wide-ranging categories as weddings, pregnancy, cooking, music instruction, foreign language, crafts, pets, New Age, and so much more. When you're done reading them all, you can finally say you know *Everything*®!

QUESTION

Answers to
common questions

FACT

Important snippets
of information

ALERT

Urgent
warnings

ESSENTIAL

Quick
handy tips

PUBLISHER Karen Cooper

DIRECTOR OF ACQUISITIONS AND INNOVATION Paula Munier

MANAGING EDITOR, EVERYTHING® SERIES Lisa Laing

COPY CHIEF Casey Ebert

ACQUISITIONS EDITOR Katrina Schroeder

DEVELOPMENT EDITOR Brett Palana-Shanahan

EDITORIAL ASSISTANT Ross Weisman

EVERYTHING® SERIES COVER DESIGNER Erin Alexander

LAYOUT DESIGNERS Colleen Cunningham, Elisabeth Lariviere, Ashley Vierra, Denise Wallace

Visit the entire Everything® series at *www.everything.com*

THE
EVERYTHING®
DIABETES
COOKBOOK
2ND EDITION

Gretchen Scalpi, RD, CDN, CDE

Foreword by C. Ranjan Nath, MD

▲adamsmedia
Avon, Massachusetts

To Jon Hines, for your wonderfully creative ideas,
great food, good times, and everlasting friendship.

An Everything® Series Book.

Everything® and everything.com® are registered trademarks of F+W Media, Inc.

Published by Adams Media, a division of F+W Media, Inc.
57 Littlefield Street, Avon, MA 02322 U.S.A.
www.adamsmedia.com

ISBN 10: 1-4405-0154-8
ISBN 13: 978-1-4405-0154-8
eISBN 10: 1-4405-0155-6
eISBN 13: 978-1-4405-0155-5

Printed in the United States of America.

10 9 8 7 6 5 4 3

Library of Congress Cataloging-in-Publication Data
is available from the publisher.

This publication is designed to provide accurate and authoritative information with regard to the subject matter covered. It is sold with the understanding that the publisher is not engaged in rendering legal, accounting, or other professional advice. If legal advice or other expert assistance is required, the services of a competent professional person should be sought.

—From a *Declaration of Principles* jointly adopted by a Committee of the American Bar Association and a Committee of Publishers and Associations

Many of the designations used by manufacturers and sellers to distinguish their products are claimed as trademarks. Where those designations appear in this book and Adams Media was aware of a trademark claim, the designations have been printed with initial capital letters.

The information contained in this book is intended to communicate information which is helpful and educational to the reader. It is not intended to replace medical diagnosis or treatment, but rather to provide information and recipes which may be helpful in implementing a diet program prescribed by your doctor. Please consult your physician for medical advice before changing your diet.

This book is available at quantity discounts for bulk purchases.
For information, please call 1-800-289-096

Contents

Acknowledgments

Thank you to the staff at Adams Media, especially Katrina Schroeder and Brett Shanahan, for their advice, encouragement, and technical support during my first journey as a cookbook author.

Thanks to all of my diabetic clients who have taught me and given me perspective about what it is like to live with diabetes.

I am deeply appreciative to my husband John, who, for thirty-six years, has always supported my career endeavors, and made my life easier during busy and stressful times.

To my husband John, son Joe, and family members Lydia, Chris, Jeff, and Haley: many thanks for your willingness to sample my many recipe "experiments" and provide much-needed feedback!

Lastly, a thank you to my parents, Marty and Jacky Sorenson, who helped me get started on what has become a very interesting and sometimes surprising career path.

Foreword

It gives me great pleasure to write a few words on *The Everything® Diabetes Cookbook, 2nd Edition*. On a personal note, I have known Gretchen Scalpi for quite some time now and have developed a collaborative working relationship with her, as she has been the main source of nutritional counseling for my patients. Most importantly, I have always received positive feedback about Gretchen from my patients, who are appreciative of her practical and easy-to-adhere-to dietary recommendations.

Type 2 Diabetes Mellitus (T2DM) presently affects over 24 million Americans, and projections suggest that the number of diabetics will double to an astounding 50 million within the next twenty-five years. Our focus as health care professionals must be to identify the condition with its initial manifestations in order to facilitate early intervention with therapeutic lifestyle changes and hopefully delay pharmacological treatment, with its inherent side effects.

Dietary management of diabetes does not mean carb abstinence, a prevailing myth. As aptly noted, it is the reduction of carbohydrates, as well as emphasizing the consumption of more complex carbs than simple sugars, that remains imperative. The section on carbs clearly distinguishes simple versus complex carbs and represents a significant point while presenting a clearer understanding to the reader. These general recommendations are both sensible and helpful hints. As a society, we tend to supersize most of our food portions; hence, I commend the emphasis on portion control that is critically important to follow on a daily basis.

Although most people think they're familiar with cholesterol/fats, in general their know-how is rather vague when it comes to differentiating saturated versus unsaturated fats; therefore, the section on fats explicitly defines the distinction between them. This is a valuable piece of information, as in recent years both the American Diabetes Association and the American Heart Association equate diabetes mellitus to coronary artery disease. In this context, nutritional management of diabetes mellitus must and should include reducing intakes of fats, specifically saturated fats.

The hallmark of this book is its simplicity—it is easy to read, easy to comprehend, and easy to execute. While there is a plethora of dietetic information accessible to the public, this book harnesses the information for daily application. Therapeutic lifestyle change means behavior modification, nutritional balance, regular exercise, and weight reduction. Not only does this book provide valuable nutritional tidbits in the management of diabetes mellitus, it offers helpful suggestions to promote a healthier lifestyle.

C. Ranjan Nath, MD

Introduction

When it comes to managing diabetes, knowledge is power. The more you know about diabetes, the better you can control it and minimize your risk of complications. Hopefully, by reading this book and putting some ideas into practice, you will have taken the first steps toward learning all you can about diabetes.

Diabetes Mellitus

For most persons with type 2 diabetes, every time you eat your body converts the foods you consume into glucose. Insulin is a hormone the body makes that enables the glucose to get into cells for use as energy. Someone with diabetes either lacks sufficient amounts of insulin or is unable to use the insulin they make. When insulin is absent or ineffective, the body is unable to get energy into cells and the level of glucose in the blood increases. Genetics, obesity, and lack of exercise appear to be causal factors in most cases of diabetes.

Type 1 Diabetes

Approximately 5–10 percent of known cases of diabetes are classified as type 1 diabetes. Type 1 diabetes was formerly referred to as juvenile-onset diabetes because the onset typically occurs before the age of thirty. Type 1 diabetes is an autoimmune disorder that is thought to develop when stress factors (such as a viral infection) damage or destroy the beta cells of the pancreas. The person with type 1 diabetes is always dependent upon insulin because their pancreas no longer produces insulin. Type 1 diabetes is usually not associated with obesity or lack of exercise.

Type 2 Diabetes

Type 2 diabetes affects the vast majority of individuals who have diabetes. For most type 2 diabetics, the pancreas still produces insulin, but it is being produced in insufficient amounts or the body is unable to use the insulin in an efficient way.

Type 2 diabetes is generally diagnosed in mid to late adulthood. Unfortunately, with the increase and prevalence of obesity among children, practitioners are now seeing children with type 2 diabetes as well.

Type 2 diabetes is usually related to a sedentary lifestyle and an overweight or obese status. If diagnosed early enough, this form of diabetes can often be controlled with weight loss, proper eating habits, and exercise. It is important to understand that diabetes is a disease that progresses, and while it can be controlled, it cannot be cured. Over time, many persons with type 2 diabetes may require oral medications and/or insulin to effectively treat and manage the disease.

Gestational Diabetes

Gestational diabetes is similar to type 2 diabetes because the body still makes insulin; however, a hormone secreted by the placenta interferes with the action of insulin. The result is elevated blood glucose levels, usually starting around the twenty-fourth to twenty-eighth week of the pregnancy. In most cases, the pregnant woman's blood glucose returns to normal after the delivery of the baby and the diabetes is gone. A woman who has had gestational diabetes in the past has an increased risk of developing type 2 diabetes later in her life.

Gestational diabetes is usually treated in a similar way to type 2 diabetes, through proper eating habits, weight control, and exercise. If blood glucose does not normalize with these measures, it may become necessary to use insulin to control the diabetes for the duration of the pregnancy. Oral diabetic medications cannot be used during pregnancy.

The major health concerns with gestational diabetes are macrosomia (a fetus that has grown too large for normal delivery) and hypoglycemia (low blood sugar) in the infant after delivery.

Summary

Careful and routine monitoring of blood glucose is extremely important for all diabetics. Activity and timing of insulin, medications, and meals must be taken into consideration to prevent highs and lows.

When blood glucose is very low (hypoglycemia), the individual may exhibit symptoms of disorientation, sweating, hunger, shakiness, pale skin color, or dizziness. If hypoglycemia occurs, the blood glucose should be tested immediately to verify a low. Hypoglycemia needs to be treated by consuming a form of carbohydrate that can get into the bloodstream quickly. All persons with diabetes and particulary those with type 1 diabetes, should understand and know how to treat hypoglycemia. One procedure for treating hypoglycemia is known as the "Rule of 15":

1. Take 15 grams of carbohydrate (4 ounces of juice or soda, 4 glucose tablets, or 5–6 Life Savers).
2. Test blood glucose in 15 minutes.
3. Treat with another 15 grams of carbohydrate if blood glucose is still low.

As you read this book, you will see the common theme of having a plan mentioned throughout. It is through planning and know-how that you will achieve optimal management of your diabetes.

CHAPTER 1

Managing Your Diabetes

Whether you have just been diagnosed with diabetes or you have dealt with it for many years, there are steps you can take to manage it effectively. A daily plan for diabetes includes a healthy eating plan, exercise, and possibly medication. Learning more about healthy eating habits and ways to prepare tasty, enjoyable foods can help you start making those changes. As you make small changes to your eating habits, you'll soon realize that you can have more control over your diabetes. Work closely with your doctor and dietitian to learn how healthy eating and lifestyle changes can make a big difference in achieving better health and better diabetes control.

Where to Start

Contrary to what you may have heard in the past, there is no strict diet you must follow. You will likely need to make some changes in your lifestyle, and sometimes changes can seem very difficult. It is usually not necessary to totally change everything about the way that you eat. Managing diabetes is more about adopting a healthier lifestyle by making small changes one at a time.

ALERT

It's very important to avoid skipping meals. Regular meal times help prevent high or low blood sugar readings. When you skip meals, you run the risk of having an unexpected low blood sugar. Skipping meals can also lead to overeating at the next meal, causing a blood sugar high.

The American Association of Diabetes Educators believes that the seven self-care behaviors shown below are effective ways to make positive changes:

1. **Eat healthy:** Make healthy food choices, understand portion sizes, and learn the best times to eat.
2. **Be active:** Include regular activity for overall fitness, weight management, and blood glucose control.
3. **Monitor:** Self-monitor your blood glucose daily to assess how food, physical activity, and medications are working.
4. **Take medication:** Understand how medications work, and when to take them.
5. **Problem solve:** Know how to problem solve. For example, a high or low blood glucose episode requires the ability to make a quick decision about food, activity, or medication.
6. **Reduce risks:** Effective risk-reduction behaviors such as smoking cessation and regular eye exams are examples of self-care that reduce risk of complications.
7. **Healthy coping**: Good coping skills that deal with the challenges of diabetes help you stay motivated to keep your diabetes in control.

There Is No Diabetic Diet

You may think that having diabetes means giving up everything you like to eat, especially carbohydrates. Nothing could be further from the truth! With the help and advice of a registered dietitian, you can adopt healthy eating habits that fit into your lifestyle. Here are several suggestions to get you started on your plan:

- Eat meals at regular intervals.
- Include nutritious snacks in your daily eating plan.
- Try new foods and experiment with whole grains, vegetables, or fruits you have never tried before.
- Work on maintaining good portion control.
- Drink plenty of water every day.

ESSENTIAL

Food portion size is critical for controlling how many calories you eat every day, and of course, for controlling your weight. If you tend to overeat at certain meals, you can start controlling portions by eating ⅓ less than you usually do. Use a smaller plate and put ⅓ less food on your plate.

Snacking is a great way to prevent excessive hunger and keep your blood sugar at a healthy level. When chosen wisely, snacks can help you work in the recommended amounts of healthful foods such as fruit or vegetables.

Trying new foods can expand the options of foods in your eating plan. Today there are many more choices of whole or minimally processed foods available to the consumer. Shopping in the produce section of the grocery store or visiting your local farmer's market can give you plenty of ideas for including some foods that you may not have used before. Large grocery stores and health food stores carry an array of different whole-grain products that, while not new, may be unfamiliar to you. Using some of the recipes in this book will introduce you to some of the lesser known but healthful whole grains.

Small Steps Every Day = Gradual Lifestyle Changes

Accept that you won't be able to change your eating habits overnight, and adopt the approach of taking small steps every day. Over time, you can make significant changes toward improving your health and reaching consistent near-normal blood glucose levels. Think of changes in your eating habits as goals rather than inflexible rules and regulations. Start by making an honest review of your current eating habits then list what you'd like to change or improve. Decide exactly how you will work on each change then select one or two changes to work on at a time. Your dietitian can help you with creative ideas for making changes. Here's an example: If you eat a candy bar as a pick-me-up late in the afternoon, try substituting a small piece of fruit and an ounce of low-fat cheese instead.

Once you've mastered a change, you can move on to something new. Some changes will be easy; others will be difficult or take more time. Start off by making easier changes first, then tackle something that would be very difficult for you.

What Can I Eat?

You may be surprised to learn that your eating plan will have the same foods that everyone else eats, and buying all sorts of specialty or diet foods is usually unnecessary. You may wish to use an artificial sweetener of your choice or certain sugar-free food items; however, this is not essential. You will not have to prepare one meal for yourself and something different for the rest of your household. As you look over the recipes in this cookbook, you will find a few specialty items, but in general the recipes use foods that everyone can eat.

Carbohydrates and Diabetes: Facts You Should Know

Carbohydrates serve as the body's primary energy source. Simple carbohydrates include all kinds of sugars, sweets, juices, and fruits. Complex carbohydrates include all types of grain products and starchy vegetables such as potatoes or corn. General recommendations for a healthy diet and your diabetes suggest that you get most of your carbohydrates in the form of complex carbohydrates rather than simple sugars. Complex carbohydrates provide an important source of vitamins, minerals, and fiber. Although fruits contain simple sugar, they are also good sources of vitamins, minerals, and fiber, and therefore should be included. To get more fiber, make most of the fruit choices in your eating plan fresh fruit rather than juice.

QUESTION

What are whole grains?
The FDA has defined whole grains as "the intact, ground, cracked or flaked fruit of the grains whose principal components—the starchy endosperm, germ and bran—are present in the same relative proportions as they exist in the intact grain." In other words, no part of the grain has been removed during the processing of the grain; you are getting all the parts of a grain.

You may be under the impression that because you have diabetes you must cut out all carbohydrates. This is definitely not the case, and you will be happy to learn there are many carbohydrate food options that you can include in your plan, as long as you choose carbohydrates that have good nutritional value and maintain an appropriate portion size.

Protein: Your Building Blocks to Good Health

Proteins are the building blocks of the body and are used for growth, building, and repair. Animal proteins such as meat, fish, eggs, and milk contain all nine essential amino acids. When all essential amino acids are present in food, it is called a complete protein.

Vegetable proteins are found in nuts, seeds, vegetables, whole grains, and legumes. All vegetable proteins, with the exception of soy, are considered incomplete proteins because one or more of the essential amino acids are missing. Even though a vegetable protein is considered incomplete, it is not considered less nutritious than a complete protein. Incomplete proteins simply need to be combined with other foods to provide the full complement of the nine essential amino acids. For example, combining rice (a grain) with beans (a legume) provides all of the essential amino acids. Combining grains, beans, nuts, vegetables, or seeds in various ways can provide a complete protein.

Fats: Poly-, Mono-, Saturated, and Trans

All fats, regardless of the type, have a significant amount of calories; therefore, moderation of any fat is your best guide. Every gram of fat contains 9 calories.

ESSENTIAL

Eating a balanced diet that includes foods from all of the essential food groups generally meets the nutrition needs of most adults. Some individuals have other health issues in addition to diabetes, and this may affect specific nutritional requirements. Discuss all of your health issues with your doctor and registered dietitian to determine whether you should take vitamin and mineral supplements or make special modifications to your diet to meet specific nutritional needs.

Monounsaturated fats should make up most of the fats you consume. This type of fat is found in certain plant foods such as walnuts, canola oil, peanut oil, or olive oil. Monounsaturated fats do not raise blood cholesterol and may actually help reduce blood cholesterol levels if they replace saturated fat in the diet.

Polyunsaturated fats should be used in moderation, and less often than monounsaturated fats. These fats come mostly from vegetable sources such as corn oil, sunflower oil, and some types of margarine.

Saturated fats should be used the least. This type of fat is typically found in foods made from animal sources such as meat, butter, cheese, or cream. Baked goods such as cakes or pastries may be high in saturated fat if lard, palm, or coconut oil is used. Excessive intake of saturated fat can increase blood cholesterol levels.

Trans fats are the result of a food manufacturing process called hydrogenation. This process converts a liquid vegetable oil to a solid fat to make shortenings and solid (stick) types of margarine.

Foods containing omega-3 fatty acids are encouraged. Omega-3 plays an important role in the maintenance of immune function, brain development, and reproduction. There is considerable evidence to suggest that omega-3 fatty acids can have a positive effect on certain conditions due to their anti-inflammatory properties. Omega-3 fatty acids are found in soy oil, green leafy vegetables, walnuts, flax seed, and most notably, oily fish such as salmon, sardines, and mackerel.

ALERT

Check food labels and ingredients to avoid trans fats as much as possible. This form of fat can raise LDL (bad) cholesterol and increase your risk for heart disease. Trans fats can be found in vegetable short-enings, solid margarines, certain crackers, cookies, and other foods made with partially hydrogenated oils.

Cholesterol

Cholesterol is a waxy substance found in all body cells. It is part of some hormones, and essential for fat digestion. The liver manufactures much of the cholesterol your body needs, but cholesterol is also obtained from the foods you eat. Cholesterol is found in animal foods such as meat, eggs, butter, and whole dairy products. Too much cholesterol in the blood can increase your risk for heart disease. People with diabetes have more risk for heart disease. It is advisable to limit consumption of fatty meats and other high-cholesterol foods to 300 milligrams or less daily. Your doctor or registered dietitian may provide you with more specific recommendations for cholesterol control.

Sodium

Sodium is a mineral that does not affect blood sugar, but it can alter your blood pressure. Controlling blood pressure is yet another important aspect of managing your diabetes. The recommended sodium intake for healthy adults is 2,400–3,000 milligrams per day. If you have high blood pressure, you may need to keep your sodium intake under 2,400 milligrams daily.

Tips for reducing sodium include:

- Leaving out or reducing the amount of salt in standard recipes by 25–50 percent
- Using commercial herb blends (or making your own) to season food instead of using salt

- Limiting intake of highly processed foods such as boxed mixes, instant foods, or processed meats
- Making more soups, stews, casseroles, or side dishes from scratch
- Watching your use of salt when cooking or at the table

About Fiber and Whole Grains

There are two types of fiber found in foods: soluble and insoluble. It's important to include foods containing both types of fiber in your daily eating plan.

Soluble fiber dissolves or swells when it's put into water. Soluble fiber helps keep blood sugar levels stable by slowing down the rate of glucose absorption into the blood stream. When consumed in adequate amounts, soluble fiber can help lower blood cholesterol levels as well. Beans, fruit, barley, and oats are especially good sources of soluble fiber.

Insoluble fiber does not dissolve in water. It is not readily broken down by bacteria in the intestinal tract, so it passes through the body. Insoluble fiber is essential for preventing constipation and diverticulosis by helping to maintain regularity. Vegetables, whole grain foods, and fruit are all good sources of insoluble fiber.

Getting More Fiber Every Day

Although all types of grains are sources of complex carbohydrates, those that have not been refined are better for you. Whole grains generally have more fiber and minerals. Because whole grains have not had the bran layer and germ removed during the milling process, fiber, as well as vitamins and minerals, are preserved. Refined grains such as white flour or white rice have the bran and germ removed—this makes the refined grain much lower in fiber. Vitamins and minerals are also removed during this process, so they must be added back into the product after processing. Adding back nutrients to a processed food is called enrichment. When you see predominant ingredients such as enriched flour in a food, odds are it has been refined and is not very high in fiber. Eating refined grains instead of whole grains makes it difficult to achieve adequate amounts of fiber each day. Whenever you can, choose whole grains over refined grains. The recommendation for daily fiber intake is 25–30 grams per day, which is about twice the amount found in the typical American diet.

FACT

Terms like "multigrain," "seven grain," or "stone ground" do not necessarily mean a product is whole grain. If a whole-grain ingredient is not listed as the first ingredient, the item may contain only a small portion of whole grains. One way to find a whole-grain product is to look for the Whole Grains Council stamp of approval, which has two different logos used to label foods containing whole grains. The logo with "100 percent Whole Grain" on it indicates the food has only whole grains and at least 16 grams per serving.

Great Ways to Get More Whole Grains

The best way to get more whole grains in your meals is to substitute whole-grain foods for refined products.

- When a recipe calls for white flour (all-purpose), experiment by replacing some of the flour with a whole-grain variety.
- Every week try one new grain. Quinoa, brown rice, bulgur, or kasha may be unfamiliar to you, but are as easy to prepare as white rice.
- Use whole grains as a side dish or mixed with vegetables, lentils, or beans.
- Add whole grains to soups, salads, or casseroles instead of white rice or pasta.
- Try a cooked whole grain as a hot breakfast cereal.
- If you are not used to bran or other high-fiber cereals, try mixing them with equal amounts of your regular cereal.
- Switch to whole-grain crackers instead of saltines or snack-type crackers.
- Use oatmeal in place of bread crumbs in items such as meatloaf or meatballs.
- Gradually start replacing the refined grains in you kitchen cabinets with whole-grain foods.

Reading and Understanding Food Labels

The nutrition facts found on food labels contain plenty of information, but unless you understand how to read the label, you may be presented with information that doesn't mean very much to you.

UNDERSTANDING TERMS ON LABELS
- **Serving size:** Each label must identify the size of a serving. The nutritional information listed on a label is based on one serving of the food. Note that the serving listed on a package may not be the same as the size of your serving.
- **Amount per serving:** Each package indentifies the quantities of nutrients and food constituents from one serving. From this information, you can find the calorie value of the food in addition to how much fat (saturated or trans), cholesterol, sodium, carbohydrates, and protein per serving.
- **Percent daily value:** This indicates how much of a specific nutrient a serving of food contains in comparison to an average 2,000-calorie diet.
- **Ingredient list:** A list of the ingredients in a food in descending order of predominance and weight.

Compare Carbohydrate Grams to Grams of Sugar

There are several parts to the carbohydrate section of the nutrition label. Total carbohydrates represent the amount of carbohydrate grams found in a food. Beneath the total carbohydrates line are other listings: fiber, sugars, and sometimes sugar alcohols. These values are part of the total carbohydrate.

ESSENTIAL

By comparing the calories from fat to the total calories in a food, you can identify foods that have lots of hidden fat. A typical hot dog has 110 total calories and 90 calories from fat. This means that 82 percent of the calories in the hot dog come from fat! Making this determination before buying a food can help you make healthier choices. Look for foods with 30 percent or less of its calories from fat.

When you look at the grams of sugars in a product, be sure to compare it to the grams of total carbohydrate. For example, if a cup of cereal has 32 grams total carbohydrate and 16 grams of sugars, that means 50 percent of the carbohydrate in the cereal comes from sugars. Try to choose foods with 30 percent or less grams of sugars.

Fiber grams are also part of the total carbohydrate. Remember that fiber helps to slow down the absorption of glucose in the bloodstream. Choose foods that contain 4 or more grams of fiber per serving.

The Glycemic Index

The glycemic index (GI) measures how a food with carbohydrate raises blood glucose. Foods are ranked on a scale from 0 to 100, based on a comparison to a reference food. Glucose is generally used as the benchmark for this comparison. A food with a high GI has more impact on blood sugar than a food with a medium or low GI.

Using the GI for meal planning involves choosing foods with a low or medium GI and limiting foods known to have a high GI. Eating foods with a lower GI can help control blood sugar and insulin levels in the body. Examples of carbohydrate foods with a low GI include dried beans and legumes, nonstarchy vegetables, most whole fruits, and many whole-grain breads and cereals. Foods that don't contain carbohydrate (such as meats or fats) do not have a GI.

Foods that are good sources of fiber tend to have a lower GI. In general, the less processed a food is, the lower the GI. The GI of a food can be affected by its degree of ripeness, the amount and type of processing it has sustained, or the method in which it has been cooked. For example, a very ripe piece of fruit will have a higher GI than one that is not as ripe. Pasta that is cooked al dente has a lower GI than soft-cooked pasta. Fruit juices, because of more processing, usually have a higher GI than fresh fruit.

When it comes to meal planning for diabetes, there is no right way that works well for everyone. The GI is one of several tools you can use in conjunction with maintaining portion control. If you choose to use the GI as a meal-planning tool, keep in mind that the total amount of carbohydrate you eat is still the most important factor. For more information about the glycemic index, go to: *www.joslin.org* or *www.mendosa.com/gilists.htm*.

Your Grocery Shopping List

Having a plan and the right foods on hand is the best way to keep you eating healthier. If you don't have a good plan and leave things to chance, you could make poor food choices. Grabbing a fast-food or take-out meal at the last minute usually means you will be eating fewer vegetables, fresh fruit, or whole-grain foods. At the same time, you will be consuming plenty of calories, fat, refined grains, and possibly sugar. Set aside some time each week to plan your meals. If you work or have a very busy schedule, a good time to plan or shop may be your day off or a quiet time of the day. A little bit of time invested in meal planning saves time and money.

Keep a weekly shopping list visible and handy; when you think of food items you need, you can write them on your list. Each time you plan, consider what meals and snacks you will need for the coming week. As you develop a shopping list, take stock of the types of foods you have in your kitchen cabinets, refrigerator, and freezer, then decide what you need to add.

Having plenty of healthy food choices available all of the time helps you avoid the pitfalls of eating too many empty-calorie foods that get in the way of weight loss or managing your diabetes.

TWENTY FOODS TO ALWAYS HAVE ON HAND
1. Vegetables: Any fresh, frozen, or reduced-sodium canned
2. Fruits: Any fresh, frozen (unsweetened), or canned (juice or water packed)
3. Whole-grain bread
4. High-fiber (low sugar) cereals with 4 grams or more fiber per serving
5. Canned beans, dry beans, or lentils—any variety
6. Boneless, skinless chicken or turkey breast
7. Egg substitutes or egg whites
8. Tuna or salmon canned in water
9. Low-fat cheese or cheese sticks—choose 1–1½ percent fat varieties
10. Nonstick cooking spray
11. Dried herbs and spices—any single varieties or mixes made without salt
12. Nonfat dry roasted or raw nuts (walnuts and almonds are good choices)
13. Noncaloric sweetener
14. Reduced-fat mayonnaise or salad dressing
15. Low-sodium chicken, vegetable, or beef broth
16. Leafy lettuce varieties or bagged salad mixes using leafy varieties

17. One or more whole grains: quinoa, amaranth, barley, bulgur, kasha, brown rice, whole-grain pasta
18. Canned tomatoes or stewed canned tomatoes
19. Fat-free yogurt—plain, vanilla, or fruit flavored, artificially sweetened
20. Whole-grain crackers

Make Over Your Food Supply

Making over your food supply does not have to be extreme, costly, or stressful. You can gradually make over your cupboards by phasing out foods of lesser nutritional quality with newer ones that have more health benefits or lower calories. As you run out of items that you already have, replace the item with something new.

▼ SUGGESTIONS FOR SWITCHING TO HEALTHIER FOODS

Instead of	Replace it with
Garlic or Onion Salt	Fresh Garlic or Onion
Fruit Juices	Fresh Fruit
All-Purpose Flour	Whole-Wheat or Rye Flour
Vegetable Oil	Olive or Canola Oil
Sour Cream	Plain Low-Fat Yogurt
Buttery Snack Crackers	Whole-Grain Crackers
Cookies	Graham Crackers
Potato Chips	Popcorn (Make Your Own)
Half Gallon of Ice Cream	Single Serving Reduced-Calorie Ice Cream
Bacon	Thin-Sliced Low-Fat Ham

Making Recipe Adjustments

Your favorite recipes can be adjusted to lower fat, salt, or sugar content, yet still maintain good taste. Recipes that are cooked rather than baked can often turn out quite well with a simple reduction in sugar, salt, or fat. It is possible to substitute low-fat or low-sodium ingredients in certain recipes. As an example, using 1% milk instead of whole milk in a pudding recipe lowers fat and calories without significantly altering the taste.

Some of the recipes found in this cookbook may contain ingredients such as butter or salt in small amounts. These ingredients are usually part of a recipe because they improve the flavor of a food or aid in the baking process. When baking bread, cookies, or cakes, salt is usually required in the leavening process and should not be eliminated. If you must eliminate all butter from your diet, most recipes can use margarine or vegetable oil as a substitute. You and your dietitian can decide whether it is appropriate to include these ingredients in small quantities or make a substitution.

QUESTION

Can sugar be eliminated from my favorite cake and cookie recipes?
Completely eliminating sugar from baked desserts can be tricky. Although sugar is an empty-calorie food, it does serve as an important ingredient in certain baked foods by enhancing the flavor, texture, or appearance. When sugar is reduced or replaced with an artificial sweetener in a cake or cookie recipe, the result can be very different. The end product can be denser, lack a golden brown color, or have a flavor unlike the original recipe.

The recipes for baked desserts found in this cookbook have different methods for addressing sugar in the recipe. Some recipes will simply have a reduction in the total amount of sugar used; others use a different type of sugar that has caloric value, such as honey or maple syrup. When these are used in the place of sugar, a lesser quantity is used; it is lower in sugar, but not sugar free. Lastly, some recipes have a combination of an artificial sweetener with a very small amount of regular sugar. As you work with these, or with your own recipes, you will learn how to adjust ingredients to get good results.

Tips for Replacing or Reducing Sugar and Fat

- Try reducing a standard recipe's sugar content 25–50 percent. It's usually best to start with a smaller reduction (25 percent) and gradually decrease the amount of sugar each time you make it. Be sure to note whether the properties of the food have any significant or undesirable changes, then adjust as needed.

- Use puréed, unsweetened fruit or fruit juices to replace some or all of the sugar in a recipe.
- Honey or maple syrup will affect blood sugar; however, either can add sweetness to a food. Carbohydrate and calories can be reduced in a recipe if you use a smaller amount of these sugars in a recipe.
- Many recipes can withstand up to a 50 percent reduction in fat. To replace fat but not volume, try using plain yogurt, applesauce, mashed ripe banana, or other puréed fruit for half of the oil or shortening called for in a recipe. If the product requires sweetness in addition to volume, applesauce or mashed ripe banana make good options.

Using Sugar Substitutes

Sugar substitutes are never mandatory for diabetes management, but they can offer options to those who may wish to use them. Using a sugar substitute in recipes can slash sugar and a significant amount of calories. When using sugar substitutes in baking, keep in mind that sweetness is being added to the food, but other traits unique to a baked product (volume, texture, golden-brown color) may be altered.

The sweeteners listed below are all approved by the FDA. They vary in taste, uses, and suitability for cooking or baking. You will need to do a taste test on your own to decide which ones are best for you.

▼ **SUGAR SUBSTITUTES**

Sweetener	Brand	Name Notes
Saccharin	Sweet N'Low or Sugar Twin	Saccharin can leave a bitter aftertaste, and may need to be combined with other sweeteners to improve taste when used in cooking. Twenty-four packets replaces 1 cup of sugar.
Aspartame	Equal, NutraSweet	High temperatures diminish sweetness, making this product less suitable for baking. Aspartame contains phenylalanine, which can be harmful to people with the rare disease Phenylketonuria (PKU).
Sucralose	Splenda	There are several baking products using sucralose, including a granular version that measures cup for cup with sugar. There are also half sugar/brown sugar blends that contain sugar, so adjust accordingly.
Stevia	Truvia, PureVia	Look for brands of stevia that use a purified portion of the stevia leaf known as rebaudioside A. Sugar-to-stevia ratios vary with each brand, so follow recommendations by the manufacturer if using in cooking or baking.

What about Alcohol?

When it comes to alcohol and diabetes management, it's all about moderation. Consider the facts about alcohol then decide whether including alcohol on a moderate basis fits into your diabetes plan. Alcohol does not provide any essential nutrients, but it is a source of calories. At 7 calories per gram, too much alcohol can promote weight gain. If you drink and are having difficulty losing weight, do not overlook the calories that alcohol adds to your overall intake. Alcohol can significantly impact blood lipid levels and elevate triglycerides; both of these health issues may already be a source of concern if you have diabetes.

FACT

If your diabetes is well controlled, you may be able to drink a moderate amount of alcohol. Moderation is considered two drinks a day for men and one drink a day for women. One drink is a 12-ounce beer, 5-ounce glass of wine, or 1½ ounces of 80-proof distilled spirits. Beverages with mixers (sodas, juices, etc.) have more carbohydrates. If you use mixers, lower the calories and carbohydrates by using club soda, mineral water, diet soda, or diet tonic water in the drink.

Alcohol prevents the liver from producing glucose. While this sounds like it could be helpful, the results can actually be quite harmful. The person who takes insulin or any diabetic medication designed to lower blood glucose may experience hypoglycemia (low blood sugar) shortly after drinking. The hypoglycemia can continue for many hours beyond that. In short, if you choose to drink alcohol, you should always limit the amount and take the alcohol with a meal to keep your blood glucose stable.

CHAPTER 2

Appetizers

Cucumber Slices with Smoked Salmon Cream

PER SERVING: Calories: 27 | Protein: 1g | Carbohydrates: .5g | Fat: 2g | Saturated Fat: 1g
Cholesterol: 7mg | Sodium: 50mg | Fiber: .07g | PCF Ratio: 17-8-75 | Exchange Approx.: ½ Fat

INGREDIENTS | **YIELDS ABOUT ½ CUP; SERVING SIZE: 1 TEASPOON**

2–3 cucumbers
1 ounce smoked salmon
8 ounces Neufchatel cheese, room temperature
½ tablespoon lemon juice
½ teaspoon freshly ground pepper
Dried dill (optional)

1. Cut cucumbers into ¼" slices. Place on paper towels to drain while you prepare salmon cream.

2. Combine smoked salmon, Neufchatel, lemon juice, and pepper in food processor; blend until smooth.

3. Fit a pastry bag with tip; spoon salmon cream into the bag. Pipe 1 teaspoon of salmon cream atop each cucumber slice. Garnish with dried dill, if desired.

Flaxseed Oil–Fortified Salsa Dip

PER SERVING: Calories: 18 | Protein: 0g | Carbohydrates: 1g | Fat: 2g | Saturated Fat: 0g
Cholesterol: 0mg | Sodium: 49mg | Fiber: 0g | PCF Ratio: 5-17-78 | Exchange Approx.: 3 servings = 1 Fat

INGREDIENTS | **YIELDS ABOUT 1 CUP; SERVING SIZE: 1 TABLESPOON**

⅛ cup flaxseed oil
½ cup mild salsa
1 teaspoon freeze-dried chives
1 teaspoon dried basil
Pinch of sea salt
¼ cup chopped onion

Blend all ingredients together in food processor or blender for a smooth dip; otherwise, mix thoroughly with a fork.

Lemon Tahini Vegetable Dip

PER SERVING: Calories: 26 | Protein: 1g | Carbohydrates: 1g | Fat: 2g | Saturated Fat: 0g
Cholesterol: 0mg | Sodium: 61mg | Fiber: 1g | PCF Ratio: 16-11-73 | Exchange Approx.: ½ Fat

INGREDIENTS	YIELDS ABOUT 5 CUPS; SERVING SIZE: 1 TABLESPOON

1 cup sesame seeds

¼ cup lemon juice

1 cup water

2 tablespoons ground flaxseed

1 teaspoon garlic powder

⅛ teaspoon cider vinegar

1 teaspoon sea salt

Put all ingredients in food processor; blend until smooth.

French Onion Soup Dip

PER SERVING: Calories: 7 | Protein: 1g | Carbohydrates: 1g | Fat: 0g | Saturated Fat: 0g | Cholesterol: 1mg
Sodium: 11mg | Fiber: 0g | PCF Ratio: 61-28-11 | Exchange Approx.: 1 Free Condiment

INGREDIENTS	YIELDS ABOUT 1¾ CUPS; SERVING SIZE: 1 TABLESPOON

1 cup chopped sweet onion

2 tablespoons reduced (double-strength) beef broth

1 tablespoon Parmesan cheese

1 cup nonfat cottage cheese

1. Put onion and beef broth in a microwave-safe dish. Cover and microwave on high 1 minute; stir. Continue to microwave on high in 30-second intervals until onion is transparent. Stir in Parmesan cheese. Set aside and allow to cool.

2. In blender, process cottage cheese until smooth. Mix into onion mixture. Serve warm or refrigerate until needed and serve cold.

Guilt-Free Flavors

Adjust the flavor of dips or spreads without adding calories by adding onion or garlic powder or your choice of herbs.

Spicy Almond Dip

PER SERVING: Calories: 23 | Protein: 1g | Carbohydrates: 1g | Fat: 2g | Saturated Fat: 0g
Cholesterol: 0mg | Sodium: 148mg | Fiber: 0g | PCF Ratio: 12-25-63 | Exchange Approx.: ½ Fat

**INGREDIENTS | YIELDS ABOUT ½ CUP;
SERVING SIZE: 1
TABLESPOON**

¼ cup ground raw almonds
2 teaspoons Worcestershire sauce
½ teaspoon honey
½ teaspoon chili powder
1 teaspoon poppy seeds
½ teaspoon onion powder
⅛ cup water
Pinch of black pepper

Put all ingredients in food processor; blend until smooth.

Easy Onion Dip

PER SERVING: Calories: 50 | Protein: 2g | Carbohydrates: 4g | Fat: 3g | Saturated Fat: 2g
Cholesterol: 10mg | Sodium: 147mg | Fiber: 8g | PCF Ratio: 17-30-53 | Exchange Approx.: ½ Fat

**INGREDIENTS | YIELDS 2 CUPS;
SERVING SIZE: 1½
TABLESPOONS**

1 cup nonfat yogurt
1 cup reduced-fat sour cream
2 tablespoons onion flakes
½ teaspoon salt
¼ teaspoon lemon pepper
1 teaspoon dill

Mix all ingredients together. Refrigerate for 2–3 hours in covered container before serving.

Horseradish Dip

PER SERVING: Calories: 12 | Protein: 1g | Carbohydrates: 1g | Fat: 1g | Saturated Fat: 0g
Cholesterol: 0mg | Sodium: 9mg | Fiber: 0g | PCF Ratio: 39-21-40 | Exchange Approx.: 1 Free Condiment

INGREDIENTS | YIELDS 1¾ CUPS; SERVING SIZE: 1 TABLESPOON

1 cup nonfat cottage cheese
1 tablespoon olive oil
½ cup nonfat plain yogurt
3 tablespoons prepared horseradish
1 teaspoon lemon juice
Optional seasonings, to taste:
　　Onion powder
　　Cumin
　　Sea salt
　　Ginger

Combine all ingredients in blender or food processor; process until smooth.

Artichoke Dip

PER SERVING: Calories: 47 | Protein: 1g | Carbohydrates: 4g | Fat: 3g | Saturated Fat: 1g
Cholesterol: 1mg | Sodium: 129mg | Fiber: 2g | PCF Ratio: 11-33-56 | Exchange Approx.: 1 Vegetable; ½ Fat

INGREDIENTS | YIELDS ABOUT 1 CUP; SERVING SIZE: 1½ TABLESPOONS

1 cup artichoke hearts, drained
1 tablespoon red onion, chopped
1 tablespoon sundried tomatoes, chopped
1 tablespoon low-fat mayonnaise
1 tablespoon reduced-fat sour cream
2 teaspoons Parmesan cheese
1 teaspoon lemon juice
½ teaspoon garlic, minced
1 tablespoon olive oil

Put all ingredients in food processor; blend until smooth. Chill before serving.

Variation

For a variation on this recipe, you can use ¼ cup roasted red peppers instead of sundried tomatoes.

Garbanzo Dip

PER SERVING: Calories: 24 | Protein: 4g | Carbohydrates: 5g | Fat: 0g | Saturated Fat: 0g
Cholesterol: 0mg | Sodium: 1mg | Fiber: 1g | PCF Ratio: 25-73-2 | Exchange Approx.: ½ Very-Lean Meat

INGREDIENTS | **YIELDS ABOUT 2 CUPS; SERVING SIZE: 1 TABLESPOON**

3 cups cooked garbanzo (or other) white beans
½ teaspoon ground cumin
1 tablespoon lemon juice
1 tablespoon parsley flakes
¼ teaspoon dried basil
1 teaspoon onion powder
¼ teaspoon garlic powder
1 tablespoon honey

Combine all ingredients in food processor or blender; process until smooth. Add 1 teaspoon of water or bean broth if you need to thin the dip.

Herbed Cheese Spread

PER SERVING: Calories: 20 | Protein: 1g | Carbohydrates: .5g | Fat: 2g | Saturated Fat: 1g | Cholesterol: 5mg
Sodium: 26mg | Fiber: 0g | PCF Ratio: 27-6-67 | Exchange Approx.: ¼ Skim Milk or 1 Free Condiment

INGREDIENTS | **YIELDS ABOUT 1 CUP; SERVING SIZE: 1 TABLESPOON**

2 teaspoons chopped fresh parsley leaves
2 teaspoons chopped fresh chives
1 teaspoon chopped fresh thyme
½ teaspoon freshly ground black pepper
½ cup nonfat cottage cheese
4 ounces Neufchatel cheese, room temperature

Place herbs in food processor; pulse until chopped. Add cheeses; process until smooth.

Toasted Nut Garnish
Herbed Cheese Spread is good on toast sprinkled with a few toasted pine nuts, sunflower seeds, sesame seeds, or other chopped nuts. Toast nuts in small skillet in single layer. Over low heat, toast until lightly golden, stirring often to prevent burning, for 3–4 minutes. Cool on paper towels.

Zesty Almond Spread

PER SERVING, without salt: Calories: 50 | Protein: 2g | Carbohydrates: 4g | Fat: 4g | Saturated Fat: 1g
Cholesterol: 0mg | Sodium: 1mg | Fiber: 1g | PCF Ratio: 11-28-61 | Exchange Approx.: 1 Fat

INGREDIENTS | YIELDS ABOUT ¼ CUP; SERVING SIZE: 1 TABLESPOON

30 unsalted almonds
2 teaspoons honey
1 teaspoon chili powder
¼ teaspoon garlic powder
Pinch of sea salt (optional)

Place all ingredients in food processor or blender; process to desired consistency.

Almond Honey Mustard

PER SERVING, without salt: | Calories: 21 | Protein: 1g | Carbohydrates: 1g | Fat: 2g | Saturated Fat: 1g
Cholesterol: 0mg | Sodium: 6mg | Fiber: 0g | PCF Ratio: 9-19-72 | Exchange Approx.: ½ Fat

INGREDIENTS | YIELDS ABOUT ½ CUP; SERVING SIZE: 1 TEASPOON

¼ cup unsalted almond butter
2 teaspoons mustard
1 teaspoon honey
2 tablespoons lemon juice
½ teaspoon garlic powder
Pinch of cumin (optional)
Pinch of sea salt (optional)

Add all ingredients to food processor or blender; process until smooth.

Gluten-Free Sesame Seed Crackers

PER SERVING: Calories: 50 | Protein: 2g | Carbohydrates: 5g | Fat: 3g | Saturated Fat: 1g
Cholesterol: 0mg | Sodium: 5mg | Fiber: 1g | PCF Ratio: 15-38-47 | Exchange Approx.: ½ Starch

INGREDIENTS | YIELDS 36 CRACKERS; SERVING SIZE: 1 CRACKER

1½ cups spelt flour

1 cup sesame seeds

¼ cup arrowroot

1 tablespoons olive or vegetable oil

3 tablespoons nonfat yogurt

¼ cup nonfat dry milk

½ teaspoon Ener-G nonaluminum baking powder

½ cup water

⅔ teaspoon sea salt (optional)

1. Preheat oven to 400°F. Mix all ingredients; add water a little at a time to form a soft, dough-like consistency. Be careful not to work the dough too much; you do not want to knead spelt flour.

2. On floured surface, use rolling pin to roll dough to ⅛" thick. Use cookie cutter to cut into shapes; place on cookie sheet treated with nonstick spray. (Or use a pizza cutter to crosscut the dough into square- or rectangular-shaped crackers.) Prick each cracker with a fork. Bake about 12 minutes, or until golden brown. Store cooled crackers in airtight container.

Asian Gingered Almonds

PER SERVING: Calories: 58 | Protein: 2g | Carbohydrates: 2g | Fat: 5g | Saturated Fat: 1g
Cholesterol: 1mg | Sodium: 44mg | Fiber: 1g | PCF Ratio: 14-12-74 | Exchange Approx.: 1½ Fats

INGREDIENTS | YIELDS 1 CUP; SERVING SIZE: 1 TABLESPOON

2 teaspoons unsalted butter

1 tablespoon Bragg's Liquid Aminos

1 teaspoon ground ginger

1 cup slivered almonds

Good Fat!
Almonds and many other nuts fall within the good fats category because they are low in unhealthy, saturated fats.

1. Preheat oven to 350°F. In microwave-safe bowl, mix butter, Bragg's Liquid Aminos, and ginger. Microwave on high 30 seconds, or until butter is melted; blend well.

2. Spread almonds on shallow baking sheet treated with nonstick spray. Bake for 12–15 minutes, or until light gold, stirring occasionally.

3. Pour seasoned butter over almonds; stir to mix. Bake for an additional 5 minutes. Store in airtight containers in cool place.

Easy Olive Spread

PER SERVING: Calories: 15 | Protein: 1g | Carbohydrates: 1g | Fat: 1g | Saturated Fat: .5g
Cholesterol: 1mg | Sodium: 56mg | Fiber: 0g | PCF Ratio: 17-19-64 | Exchange Approx.: 1 Free Condiment

INGREDIENTS | YIELDS ABOUT 3 CUPS; SERVING SIZE: 1 TABLESPOON

1 cup black olives

3 cloves garlic

1 tablespoon fresh Italian flat-leaf parsley

1 tablespoon fresh basil

2 teaspoons minced lemon zest

Freshly ground black pepper, to taste

½ cup nonfat cottage cheese

2 tablespoons cream cheese

1 tablespoon real mayonnaise

1. Combine olives, garlic, parsley, basil, lemon zest, and black pepper in food processor; pulse until chopped. Transfer to a bowl and set aside.

2. Add cottage cheese, cream cheese, and mayonnaise to blender or food processor; process until smooth. Fold cheese mixture into chopped olive mixture.

Delicious Substitutions

Substitute marinated mushrooms or artichoke hearts for olives in this recipe.

Almond Spread

PER SERVING, without salt: Calories: 30 | Protein: 1g | Carbohydrates: 3g | Fat: 2g
Saturated Fat: 0g | Cholesterol: 0mg | Sodium: 1mg | Fiber: 1g | PCF Ratio: 11-34-56 | Exchange Approx.: ½ Fat

INGREDIENTS | YIELDS ½ CUP; SERVING SIZE: 1 TABLESPOON

¼ cup ground raw almonds

2 teaspoons honey

4 teaspoons water

Pinch of salt (optional)

In blender, combine all ingredients; process until smooth.

Toasted Almond Seasoning

Add an extra flavor dimension to salads, rice dishes, or vegetables by sprinkling toasted almonds over the top. Toast ½ cup ground raw almonds in nonstick skillet over low heat, stirring frequently until they are a light brown color. Store cooled almonds in airtight container in cool, dry place. This low-sodium substitute has only 16 calories per teaspoon, a PCF Ratio of 14-12-74, and counts as ½ Fat Exchange Approximation.

Garlic and Feta Cheese Dip

PER SERVING: Calories: 11 | Protein: 0g | Carbohydrates: 0g | Fat: 1g | Saturated Fat: 1g | Cholesterol: 0mg
Sodium: 22mg | Fiber: 0g | PCF Ratio: 9-10-80 | Exchange Approx.: 1 Free Condiment

**INGREDIENTS | YIELDS 1½ CUPS;
SERVING SIZE: 1
TABLESPOON**

½ cup feta cheese, crumbled

4 ounces softened cream cheese

¼ cup real mayonnaise

1 clove dry-roasted garlic

¼ teaspoon dried basil

¼ teaspoon dried cilantro or oregano

⅛ teaspoon dried dill

⅛ teaspoon dried thyme

In food processor, combine all ingredients; process until thoroughly mixed. Cover and chill until ready to serve with assorted vegetables.

This dip is somewhat high in fat if you use regular cream cheese, whereas nonfat cream cheese would lower the total fat in this recipe by 38 grams. People on a salt-restricted diet need to check with their dietitians about using nonfat cream cheese because it's much higher in sodium.

Dry-Roasted Garlic

To dry-roast garlic: Preheat oven to 350°F; lightly spray small, covered baking dish with nonstick spray. Slice off ½" from top of each garlic head; rub off any loose skins, being careful not to separate cloves. Place in baking dish, cut-side up (if roasting more than 1 head, arrange in dish so they don't touch). Cover and bake until the garlic cloves are very tender when pierced, about 30–45 minutes. Roasted garlic heads will keep in refrigerator 2–3 days.

Herbed Yogurt Cheese Spread

PER SERVING: Calories: 36 | Protein: 4g | Carbohydrates: 5g | Fat: 0g | Saturated Fat: 0g
Cholesterol: 1mg | Sodium: 146mg | Fiber: 0g | PCF Ratio: 41-56-3 | Exchange Approx.: ½ Milk

INGREDIENTS | SERVING SIZE: 4 TABLESPOONS

1½ cups plain nonfat yogurt

1 tablespoon scallion, minced

1 tablespoon parsley, minced

1 teaspoon garlic, minced

2 tablespoons roasted red pepper, minced

¼ teaspoon salt

Pinch of cayenne

1. Prepare yogurt cheese in advance: Line fine mesh strainer with a coffee filter. Place plain yogurt in filter; set strainer over a bowl. Cover and refrigerate for 8 hours or overnight. When all fluid has drained, it should be consistency of softened cream cheese.

2. Add scallions, parsley, garlic, red pepper, salt, and cayenne. Mix well and refrigerate.

3. Serve with crackers or raw vegetables.

Get Your Calcium!

Yogurt is one of the top sources of calcium, a vital mineral for bone health. Yogurt cheese is very easy to make and can often be substituted in dip (or other) recipes that call for cream cheese. Cream cheese, unlike yogurt, contains mostly fat and is not a significant source of calcium or protein.

Mushroom Caviar

PER SERVING: Calories: 9 | Protein: 0g | Carbohydrates: 1g | Fat: 1g | Saturated Fat: 0g
Cholesterol: 0mg | Sodium: 1mg | Fiber: 0g | PCF Ratio: 11-32-57 | Exchange Approx.: 1 Free Condiment

INGREDIENTS | YIELDS ABOUT 3 CUPS; SERVING SIZE: 1 TABLESPOON

1½ cups portobello mushrooms

1½ cups white button mushrooms

¼ cup chopped scallions

4 cloves dry-roasted garlic (see page 26)

1 teaspoon fresh lemon juice

½ teaspoon balsamic vinegar

1 tablespoon extra-virgin olive oil

½ teaspoon fresh chopped thyme (optional)

Sea salt and freshly ground black pepper, to taste (optional)

1. Cut portobello mushrooms into ¼" cubes. Cut white button mushrooms into halves or quarters. (The mushroom pieces should be roughly uniform in size.) Place mushrooms and chopped scallion in microwave-safe bowl; cover and microwave on high 1 minute. Rotate bowl; microwave in 30-second intervals until tender.

2. Transfer scallions and mushrooms to food processor. (Reserve any liquid to use for thinning, if necessary.) Pulse several times to chop mixture, scraping down sides of bowl as needed. Add remaining ingredients; pulse until mixed. Place in small crock or serving bowl; serve warm with toasted bread. Refrigerated leftovers will last a few days.

Pseudo-Sauté

When onions and scallions are sautéed in butter or oil, they go through a caramelization process that doesn't occur when they're steamed. To create this flavor without increasing fat in a recipe, transfer steamed vegetables to a nonstick wok or skillet (coated with nonstick spray, or a small portion of oil called for in recipe) and sauté until extra moisture evaporates.

CHAPTER 3

Soups

Cold Roasted Red Pepper Soup

PER SERVING, without salt: Calories: 73 | Protein: 5g | Carbohydrates: 9g | Fat: 4g | Saturated Fat: 1g
Cholesterol: 3mg | Sodium: 404mg | Fiber: 3g | PCF Ratio: 21-39-40 | Exchange Approx.: ½ Fat, ½ Starch

INGREDIENTS | SERVES 4

1 teaspoon olive oil

½ cup chopped onion

3 roasted red bell peppers, seeded and chopped (see page 196)

3¼ cups low-fat, reduced-sodium chicken broth

½ cup nonfat plain yogurt

½ teaspoon sea salt (optional)

4 sprigs fresh basil (optional)

1. Heat saucepan over medium-high heat. Add olive oil; sauté onion until transparent. Add peppers and broth. Bring to a boil; reduce heat and simmer for 15 minutes. Remove from heat; purée in blender or food processor until smooth.

2. Allow to cool. Stir in yogurt and salt, if using; chill well in refrigerator. Garnish the soup with fresh basil sprigs, if desired.

Lentil-Vegetable Soup

PER SERVING, with water: Calories: 273 | Protein: 16g | Carbohydrates: 53g | Fat: 1g | Saturated Fat: 0g
Cholesterol: 0mg | Sodium: 34mg | Fiber: 19g | PCF Ratio: 23-74-3 | Exchange Approx.: 1 Very-Lean Meat,
3 Starches, 1 Vegetable

INGREDIENTS | SERVES 4

5 cups water or your choice of broth

1 medium-sized sweet potato, peeled and chopped

1 cup uncooked lentils

2 medium onions, chopped

¼ cup barley

2 tablespoons parsley flakes

2 carrots, sliced

1 celery stalk, chopped

2 teaspoons cumin

Combine all ingredients in soup pot; simmer until lentils are soft, about 1 hour.

Fresh Tomato Basil Soup

PER SERVING: Calories: 87 | Protein: 3g | Carbohydrates: 12g | Fat: 4g | Saturated Fat: 2g
Cholesterol: 10mg | Sodium: 449mg | Fiber: 3g | PCF Ratio: 13-50-37 | Exchange Approx.: 2 Vegetables, 1 Fat

INGREDIENTS | SERVES 6

1 tablespoon butter

¼ cup onion, chopped

4 cups (2 pounds) crushed tomatoes

¼ cup fresh basil leaves, loosely chopped

1 cup low-sodium chicken broth

2 ounces reduced fat (Neufchatel) cream cheese

Fresh ground pepper, to taste

1. Melt butter in soup pot. Add onions; sauté until soft. Add crushed tomato, basil, and chicken broth.

2. Bring to a boil. Reduce heat; cook for another 15 minutes. Remove from heat; stir in cream cheese until melted.

3. Transfer to food processor or blender; purée until smooth. Depending on size of processor or blender, you may need to purée a partial portion at a time.

Lentil Soup with Herbs and Lemon

PER SERVING: Calories: 214 | Protein: 15g | Carbohydrates: 34g | Fat: 3g | Saturated Fat: 1g | Cholesterol: 0mg
Sodium: 353mg | Fiber: 16g | PCF Ratio: 27-61-12 | Exchange Approx.: 1 Lean Meat, 2 Starches, 1 Vegetable

INGREDIENTS | SERVES 4

1 cup lentils, soaked overnight in 1 cup water

6 cups low-fat, reduced-sodium chicken broth

1 carrot, sliced

1 stalk celery, sliced

1 yellow onion, thinly sliced

2 teaspoons olive oil

1 tablespoon dried tarragon

½ teaspoon dried oregano

Sea salt and black pepper, to taste (optional)

1 tablespoon lemon juice

4 thin slices of lemon

1. Drain and rinse lentils. Add lentils and broth to pot over medium heat; bring to a boil. Reduce heat and simmer until tender, approximately 15 minutes. (If you did not presoak the lentils, increase cooking time by about 15 more minutes.)

2. While lentils are cooking, sauté carrot, celery, and onion in oil for 8 minutes, or until onion is golden brown. Remove from heat and set aside.

3. When lentils are tender, add vegetables, tarragon, oregano, and salt and pepper, if using; cook for 2 minutes. Stir in lemon juice. Ladle into 4 serving bowls; garnish with lemon slices.

Tomato-Vegetable Soup

PER SERVING: Calories: 158 | Protein: 5g | Carbohydrates: 31g | Fat: 3g | Saturated Fat: 1g | Cholesterol: 0mg
Sodium: 349mg | Fiber: 5g | PCF Ratio: 12-72-16 | Exchange Approx.: 1½ Starches, 1 Vegetable

INGREDIENTS | SERVES 6

1 tablespoon olive oil

2 teaspoons minced garlic

⅔ teaspoon cumin

2 carrots, chopped

2 stalks celery, diced

1 medium onion, chopped

⅔ cup unsalted tomato paste

½ teaspoon red pepper flakes

2 cups canned unsalted peeled tomatoes, with juice

⅔ teaspoon chopped fresh oregano

3 cups low-fat, reduced-sodium chicken broth

3 cups fat-free beef broth

2 cups diced potatoes

2 cups shredded cabbage

½ cup green beans

½ cup fresh or frozen corn kernels

½ teaspoon freshly cracked black pepper

¼ cup lime juice or balsamic vinegar

1. Heat olive oil in large stockpot; sauté garlic, cumin, carrot, and celery 1 minute. Add onion; cook until transparent.

2. Stir in tomato paste; sauté until it begins to brown.

3. Add remaining ingredients except for lime juice or vinegar. Bring to a boil; reduce heat and simmer for 20–30 minutes, adding additional broth or water if needed. Just before serving, add lime juice or balsamic vinegar.

Easy Measures

Consider freezing broth in an ice cube tray. Most ice cube tray sections hold ⅛ cup (2 tablespoons) of liquid. Once broth is frozen, you can transfer cubes to freezer bag or container. This makes it easy to measure out the amount you need for recipes.

Nutty Greek Snapper Soup

PER SERVING: Calories: 309 | Protein: 39g | Carbohydrates: 25g | Fat: 6g | Saturated Fat: 1g | Cholesterol: 46mg
Sodium: 240mg | Fiber: 2g | PCF Ratio: 50-33-17 | Exchange Approx.: 4 Lean Meats, 1 Skim Milk, 1 Vegetable

INGREDIENTS | SERVES 4

1 pound (16 ounces) red snapper fillet

2 large cucumbers

4 green onions, chopped

4 cups nonfat plain yogurt

1 cup packed fresh parsley, basil, cilantro, arugula, and chives, mixed

3 tablespoons lime juice

Salt and pepper, to taste (optional)

¼ cup chopped walnuts

Herb sprigs for garnish (optional)

Tip

You can make this soup using leftover fish or substitute halibut, cod, or sea bass for the snapper.

1. Rinse red snapper fillet and pat dry with paper towels. Broil fillet until opaque through the thickest part, about 4 minutes on each side depending on the thickness of fillet. Let cool. (Alternatives would be to steam or poach the fillets.)

2. Peel and halve cucumbers and scoop out and discard seeds; cut into 1" pieces. Put half of cucumber with green onions in bowl of food processor; pulse to coarsely chop. Transfer to a large bowl.

3. Add remaining cucumber, yogurt, and herb leaves to food processor; process until smooth and frothy. (Alternatively, you can grate cucumbers, finely mince green onion and herbs, and stir together with yogurt in large bowl.) Stir in lime juice and season with salt and pepper to taste, if using. Cover and refrigerate for at least 1 hour, or up to 8 hours; the longer the soup cools, the more the flavors will mellow.

4. While soup cools, break cooled red snapper fillet into large chunks, discarding skin and any bones. Ladle chilled soup into shallow bowls and add red snapper. Sprinkle chopped walnuts over soup, garnish with herb sprigs, and serve.

Minestrone Soup Genoese Style

PER SERVING: Calories: 201 | Protein: 9g | Carbohydrates: 29g | Fat: 6g | Saturated Fat: 2g | Cholesterol: 5mg
Sodium: 271mg | Fiber: 6g | PCF Ratio: 17-56-27 | Exchange Approx.: 1½ Starches, 1 Vegetable, 1 Fat

INGREDIENTS | SERVES 6

4 cloves garlic, minced

2 tablespoons basil, chopped

¼ teaspoon salt

2 tablespoons olive oil

1 ounce Romano cheese

2 cups cabbage, shredded

1 cup zucchini, diced

1 cup green beans, cut into 1" pieces

1 cup potatoes, peeled and chopped

2 cups navy beans, cooked

½ cup celery, chopped

¼ cup peas, fresh or frozen

1 tablespoon tomato paste

3 cups water

Salt and pepper, to taste

1. Combine garlic, basil, and salt. Add olive oil and Romano cheese; mix well into a paste and set aside. (Using a mortar and pestle works very well.)

2. Combine cabbage, zucchini, green beans, potatoes, cooked navy beans, celery, peas, tomato paste, and water in a 4–6 quart soup pot.

3. Bring to a boil; reduce heat and simmer for 45–60 minutes, or until tender.

4. Mix garlic paste into soup; simmer an additional 5 minutes. Serve.

Tip

Make extra garlic paste (using first 5 ingredients and step 1) and keep refrigerated. You'll have instant garlic-cheese flavor on hand for soups, sauces, garlic bread, and pasta dishes. Garlic paste keeps in the refrigerator for up to 2 weeks.

Broccoli and Whole-Grain Pasta Soup

PER SERVING: Calories: 86 | Protein: 6g | Carbohydrates: 10g | Fat: 3g | Saturated Fat: 1g | Cholesterol: 9mg
Sodium: 185mg | Fiber: 2g | PCF Ratio: 25-43-32 | Exchange Approx.: ½ Starch, 1 Vegetable, 1 Fat

INGREDIENTS | SERVES 6

1–3 slices bacon, cut into 1" pieces

1 tablespoon onion, chopped

2 cloves garlic, minced

1 tablespoon tomato paste

3 cups water

1 cup eggplant, peeled and cubed

¾ teaspoon salt

¼ teaspoon pepper

½ teaspoon oregano

8 ounces broccoli florets

1 cup whole-grain pasta shells, cooked al dente

1 ounce Romano cheese, grated

1. Place bacon, onion, and garlic in a 4-quart soup pot; brown.

2. Add tomato paste, water, eggplant, salt, pepper, and oregano. Bring to a boil; reduce heat and simmer for 20 minutes, or until eggplant is soft cooked.

3. Add broccoli florets; simmer for 5 minutes, until broccoli is tender but still slightly crisp. Add cooked pasta.

4. Serve soup immediately with a sprinkling of grated cheese.

White Bean and Escarole Soup

PER SERVING: Calories: 163 | Protein: 11g | Carbohydrates: 27g | Fat: 2g | Saturated Fat: 0g | Cholesterol: 7mg
Sodium: 349mg | Fiber: 9g | PCF Ratio: 26-64-10 | Exchange Approx.: 1½ Starches, ½ Vegetable,
1½ Very-Lean Meats, 2 Fats

INGREDIENTS | SERVES 6

1 cup dry navy beans

3 cups water

1 cup onion, chopped

½ cup potato, peeled and chopped

1 clove garlic, minced

3 ounces Canadian bacon, cut in ½"
cubes

2½ cups water

¼ teaspoon pepper

½ teaspoon salt

1 teaspoon vegetable oil

8 ounces escarole, coarsely chopped

1. Place dry beans and 3 cups of water in medium saucepan. Bring to a boil; remove from heat. Allow beans to soak several hours or overnight.

2. Drain beans; place in pressure cooker with onion, potatoes, garlic, Canadian bacon, 2½ cups water, salt, pepper, and vegetable oil. Close cover securely, place pressure regulator on vent pipe, and cook for 30 minutes with pressure regulator rocking slowly. (If using an electric pressure cooker, follow manufacturer instructions.) Let pressure drop on its own.

3. Add chopped escarole; simmer for 5–10 minutes, until escarole is wilted and cooked tender.

Slow-Cooker Method

This soup can also be prepared using a slow cooker. Soak beans as described in step 1; drain. Add beans, onion, potatoes, garlic, Canadian bacon, and 2½ cups water to slow cooker. Cook for 8–10 hours. At end of cooking, add escarole; simmer for 5–10 minutes, until escarole is wilted and tender. Add salt and pepper to taste.

Winter Squash and Red Pepper Soup

PER SERVING: Calories: 137 | Protein: 3g | Carbohydrates: 24g | Fat: 3g | Saturated Fat: 1g | Cholesterol: 0mg
Sodium: 445mg | Fiber: 6g | PCF Ratio: 10-70-20 | Exchange Approx.: 1 Starch, 1 Vegetable, ½ Fat

INGREDIENTS | SERVES 6

3½ cups winter squash, cooked

1 tablespoon olive oil

1 cup onions, chopped

1 tablespoon garlic, chopped

4 ounces roasted red pepper

3 cups low-sodium chicken broth

½ cup dry white wine

2 teaspoons sugar

1 teaspoon cinnamon

½ teaspoon ginger

1 tablespoon reduced-fat sour cream (optional)

1. Wash and cut squash in half; core out seeds. Place face down on oiled 9" × 13" glass baking dish; bake at 400°F for 50–60 minutes, or until squash is cooked tender. When cool enough to handle, scoop squash out of shells and set aside.

2. In large nonstick skillet, heat olive oil. Add onions and garlic; sauté until tender and continue to cook until the onions are soft and have turned brown (caramelized).

3. Add roasted pepper and chicken broth; simmer for another 16 minutes.

4. Add cooked winter squash, white wine, sugar, cinnamon, and ginger; simmer for another 5 minutes.

5. Transfer to food processor or blender; purée until smooth. Depending on size of processor or blender, you may need to purée a partial portion at a time. If desired, stir in reduced-fat sour cream and serve.

Vegetable and Bean Chili

PER SERVING: Calories: 205 | Protein: 12g | Carbohydrates: 35g | Fat: 3g | Saturated Fat: 1g | Cholesterol: 0mg
Sodium: 156mg | Fiber: 13g | PCF Ratio: 22-65-13 | Exchange Approx.: 1 Lean Meat, 2 Starches, 1 Vegetable

INGREDIENTS | SERVES 8

4 teaspoons olive oil

2 cups cooking onions, chopped

½ cup green bell pepper, chopped

3 cloves garlic, chopped

1 small jalapeño pepper, finely chopped
(include the seeds if you like the chili
extra hot)

1 tablespoon chili powder

1 teaspoon ground cumin

1 (28-ounce) can unsalted tomatoes,
chopped and undrained

2 zucchinis, peeled and chopped

2 (15-ounce) cans unsalted kidney beans,
rinsed

1 tablespoon chopped semisweet
chocolate

3 tablespoons chopped fresh cilantro

1. Heat heavy pot over moderately high heat. Add olive oil, onions, bell pepper, garlic, and jalapeño; sauté until vegetables are softened, about 5 minutes. Add chili powder and cumin; sauté for 1 minute, stirring frequently to mix well.

2. Add tomatoes with juice and zucchini; bring to a boil. Lower heat and simmer, partially covered, for 15 minutes, stirring occasionally.

3. Stir in beans and chocolate; simmer, stirring occasionally, for additional 5 minutes, or until beans are heated through and chocolate is melted. Stir in cilantro, and serve.

Rich and Creamy Sausage-Potato Soup

PER SERVING: Calories: 326 | Protein: 17g | Carbohydrates: 53g | Fat: 6g | Saturated Fat: 2g | Cholesterol: 19mg
Sodium: 259mg | Fiber: 3g | PCF Ratio: 20-64-16 | Exchange Approx.: 1 Fat, ½ Medium-Fat Meat, 1 Starch,
1½ Skim Milks, 1 Vegetable

INGREDIENTS | SERVES 2

1 teaspoon olive oil

½ teaspoon butter

½ cup chopped onion, steamed

1 clove dry roasted garlic (page 26)

1 ounce crumbled cooked Mock Chorizo
(page 62 or 63)

¼ teaspoon celery seed

2 Yukon gold potatoes, peeled and
diced into 1" pieces

½ cup fat-free chicken broth

1½ cups Mock Cream (page 183)

1 teaspoon white wine vinegar

1 teaspoon vanilla extract

Optional seasonings to taste:

    Fresh parsley

    Sea salt and freshly ground black
    pepper

1. In saucepan, heat olive oil and butter over medium heat. Add onion, roasted garlic, chorizo, celery seed, and potatoes; sauté until heated.

2. Add chicken broth; bring to a boil. Cover saucepan, reduce heat, and maintain simmer for 10 minutes, or until potatoes are tender. Add Mock Cream and heat.

3. Remove pan from burner and stir in vinegar and vanilla.

Skim the Fat

You can remove fat from soups and stews by dropping ice cubes into the pot. The fat will cling to the cubes as you stir. Be sure to take out the cubes before they melt. Fat also clings to lettuce leaves; simply sweep them over the top of the soup. Discard ice cubes or leaves when done.

Chicken Corn Chowder

PER SERVING: Calories: 193 | Protein: 17g | Carbohydrates: 21g | Fat: 5g | Saturated Fat: 3g | Cholesterol: 39mg
Sodium: 155mg | Fiber: 2g | PCF Ratio: 22-36-42 | Exchange Approx.: 1½ Very-Lean Meats, ½ Starch,
1 Vegetable, ½ Skim Milk, ½ High-Fat Meat

INGREDIENTS | SERVES 10

1 pound boneless, skinless chicken breast, cut into chunks

1 medium onion, chopped

1 red bell pepper, diced

1 large potato, diced

2 (16-ounce) cans low-fat, reduced-sodium chicken broth

1 (8¾-ounce) can unsalted cream-style corn

½ cup all-purpose flour

2 cups skim milk

4 ounces Cheddar cheese, diced

½ teaspoon sea salt

Freshly ground pepper, to taste

½ cup processed bacon bits

1. Spray large soup pot with nonstick cooking spray; heat on medium setting until hot. Add chicken, onion, and bell pepper; sauté over medium heat until chicken is browned and vegetables are tender. Stir in potatoes and broth; bring to a boil. Reduce heat and simmer, covered, for 20 minutes. Stir in corn.

2. Blend flour and milk in bowl; gradually stir into pot. Increase heat to medium; cook until mixture comes to a boil, then reduce heat and simmer until soup is thickened, stirring constantly. Add cheese; stir until melted and blended in. Add salt and pepper to taste and sprinkle with bacon bits before serving.

Tip

To trim down the fat in this recipe, use a reduced-fat cheese, such as Cabot's 50 Percent Light Cheddar.

Salmon Chowder

PER SERVING: Calories: 364 | Protein: 20g | Carbohydrates: 61g | Fat: 6g | Saturated Fat: 2g
Cholesterol: 28mg | Sodium: 199mg | Fiber: 7g | PCF Ratio: 22-65-14 | Exchange Approx.: ½ Fat,
2 Starches, 2 Lean Meats, 2 Vegetables, ½ Skim Milk

INGREDIENTS | SERVES 4

1 (7½-ounce) can unsalted salmon

2 teaspoons butter

1 medium onion, chopped

2 stalks celery, chopped

1 sweet green pepper, seeded and chopped

1 clove garlic, minced

4 carrots, peeled and diced

4 small potatoes, peeled and diced

1 cup fat-free chicken broth

1 cup water

½ teaspoon cracked black pepper

½ teaspoon dill seed

1 cup diced zucchini

1 cup Mock Cream (page 183)

1 (8¾-ounce) can unsalted cream-style corn

Freshly ground black pepper, to taste

½ cup chopped fresh parsley (optional)

1. Drain and flake salmon; discard liquid.

2. In large nonstick saucepan, melt butter over medium heat; sauté onion, celery, green pepper, garlic, and carrots, stirring often, until tender, about 5 minutes.

3. Add potatoes, broth, water, pepper, and dill seed; bring to boil. Reduce heat, cover, and simmer for 20 minutes, or until potatoes are tender.

4. Add zucchini; simmer, covered, for another 5 minutes.

5. Add salmon, Mock Cream, corn, and pepper; cook over low heat just until heated through. Just before serving, add parsley, if desired.

CHAPTER 4

Breakfast and Brunch

Buckwheat Pancakes

PER SERVING: Calories: 220 | Protein: 11g | Carbohydrates: 44g | Fat: 1g | Saturated Fat: 0g | Cholesterol: 1mg
Sodium: 200mg | Fiber: 5g | PCF Ratio: 76-19-5 | Exchange Approx.: 2 Starches, ½ Skim Milk, ½ Fruit

INGREDIENTS | SERVES 2

1 cup whole-wheat flour

½ cup buckwheat flour

1½ teaspoons baking powder

2 egg whites

¼ cup apple juice concentrate

1¼ to 1½ cups skim milk

1. Sift flours and baking powder together. Combine egg whites, apple juice concentrate, and 1¼ cups milk. Add milk mixture to dry ingredients; mix well, but do not over mix. Add remaining milk if necessary to reach desired consistency.

2. Cook pancakes in nonstick skillet or on griddle treated with nonstick spray over medium heat.

Egg White Pancakes

PER SERVING: Calories: 197 | Protein: 13g | Carbohydrates: 31g | Fat: 3g | Saturated Fat: 1g | Cholesterol: 0mg
Sodium: 120mg | Fiber: 4g | PCF Ratio: 27-61-12 | Exchange Approx.: 1 Free Sweet, 1 Lean Meat, 1½ Breads

INGREDIENTS | SERVES 2

4 egg whites

½ cup oatmeal

4 teaspoons reduced-calorie or low-sugar strawberry jam

1 teaspoon powdered sugar

1. Put all ingredients in blender; process until smooth.

2. Preheat nonstick pan treated with cooking spray over medium heat. Pour half of mixture into pan; cook for 4–5 minutes.

3. Flip pancake and cook until inside is cooked. Repeat using remaining batter for second pancake. Dust each pancake with powdered sugar, if using.

Creative Toppings

Experiment with toast and pancake toppings. Try a tablespoon of raisins, almonds, apples, bananas, berries, nut butters (limit these to 1 teaspoon per serving), peanuts, pears, walnuts, or wheat germ.

Buttermilk Pancakes

PER SERVING: Calories: 143 | Protein: 6g | Carbohydrates: 26g | Fat: 2g | Saturated Fat: 1g
Cholesterol: 49mg | Sodium: 111mg | Fiber: 1g | PCF Ratio: 16-74-10 | Exchange Approx.: 1½ Starches

INGREDIENTS | SERVES 2

1 cup all-purpose flour
2 tablespoons nonfat buttermilk powder
¼ teaspoon baking soda
½ teaspoon low-salt baking powder
1 cup water

Nut Butter Batter

For a change of pace, try adding 1
Exchange amount per serving of nut butter
to pancake batter and use jelly or jam
instead of syrup.

1. Blend together all ingredients, adding more water if necessary to get batter consistency desired.

2. Pour ¼ of batter into nonstick skillet or skillet treated with nonstick cooking spray. Cook over medium heat until bubbles appear on top half of pancake. Flip and continue cooking until center of pancake is done. Repeat process with remaining batter.

Country-Style Omelet

PER SERVING: Calories: 253 | Protein: 17g | Carbohydrates: 7g | Fat: 17g | Saturated Fat: 5g | Cholesterol: 493mg
Sodium: 221mg | Fiber: 2g | PCF Ratio: 27-12-61 | Exchange Approx.: 1 Vegetable, 2 Medium-Fat Meats, 3 Fats

INGREDIENTS | SERVES 2

2 teaspoons olive oil
1 cup zucchini, diced
¼ cup red pepper, diced
1 cup plum tomatoes, skinned and cubed
⅛ teaspoon pepper
4 eggs
1 tablespoon Parmesan cheese
1 teaspoon fresh basil, minced

1. Heat oil in nonstick skillet. Add zucchini and red pepper; sauté for 5 minutes.

2. Add tomatoes and pepper; cook uncovered for another 10 minutes, allowing fluid from tomatoes to cook down.

3. In small bowl, whisk together eggs, Parmesan cheese, and fresh basil; pour over vegetables in skillet.

4. Cook over low heat until browned, approximately 10 minutes on each side.

Fruit Smoothie

PER SERVING: The Nutritional Analysis and Fruit Exchange for this recipe will depend on your choice of fruit. Otherwise, allow ½ Skim Milk Exchange and ½ Misc. Food Exchange. The wheat germ adds fiber, but at less than 20 calories a serving, it can count as 1 Free Exchange.

INGREDIENTS | SERVES 1

1 cup skim milk
2 Exchange servings of any diced fruit
1 tablespoon honey
4 teaspoons toasted wheat germ
6 large ice cubes

Put all ingredients into blender or food processor; process until thick and smooth.

Batch 'Em

Make large batches of smoothies so you can keep single servings in the freezer. Get out a serving as you begin to get ready for your day. This should give the smoothie time to thaw enough for you to stir it when you're ready to have breakfast.

Yogurt Fruit Smoothie

PER SERVING: Calories: 149 | Protein: 10g | Carbohydrates: 26g | Fat: 1g | Saturated Fat: 0g
Cholesterol: 2mg | Sodium: 96mg | Fiber: 2g | PCF Ratio: 25-67-8 | Exchange Approx.: 1 Milk, 1 Fruit

INGREDIENTS | SERVES 2

1 cup plain low-fat yogurt
½ cup sliced strawberries
½ cup orange juice
½ cup nectarines, peeled and sliced
2 tablespoons ground flax seed

Put all ingredients in blender; process until smooth.

Variations and Combos

You can vary this smoothie by substituting other fruits of your choice. Good combinations are strawberry and banana, strawberry and kiwi, or banana and peach. Keep portions of each fruit to no more than ½ cup.

Tofu Smoothie

PER SERVING: Calories: 289 | Protein: 20g | Carbohydrates: 35g | Fat: 11g | Saturated Fat: 2g | Cholesterol: 0mg
Sodium: 19mg | Fiber: 8g | PCF Ratio: 25-44-31 | Exchange Approx.: 1 Meat Substitute, 2 Fruits

INGREDIENTS | SERVES 1

1⅓ cups frozen unsweetened strawberries

½ banana

½ cup (4 ounces) silken tofu

In food processor or blender, process all ingredients until smooth. Add a little chilled water for thinner smoothies if desired.

Overnight Oatmeal

PER SERVING: Calories: 221 | Protein: 9g | Carbohydrates: 42g | Fat: 3g | Saturated Fat: 1g | Cholesterol: 1mg
Sodium: 25mg | Fiber: 6g | PCF Ratio: 15-73-11 | Exchange Approx.: 1 Fruit, 1 Starch, ½ Skim Milk

INGREDIENTS | SERVES 4

1 cup steel-cut oats

14 dried apricot halves

1 dried fig

2 tablespoons golden raisins

4 cups water

½ cup Mock Cream (page 183)

Add all ingredients to slow cooker with a ceramic interior; set to low heat. Cover and cook overnight (8–9 hours).

Another Overnight Method

For another way to cook steel-cut oats, place 1 cup steel cut oats, 4 cups water, and dried fruit in medium saucepan; bring to a quick boil. Turn off the heat and cover saucepan. When cooled, place in covered container and refrigerate overnight. In morning, the oatmeal will have absorbed all of the water. Scoop 1 portion of the oatmeal into a bowl; microwave on high for 1½ to 2 minutes. Add milk and serve. Heat up refrigerated leftover portions as needed; use within 3 days.

Berry Puff Pancakes

PER SERVING: Calories: 110 | Protein: 5g | Carbohydrates: 37g | Fat: 2g | Saturated Fat: 1g
Cholesterol: 71mg | Sodium: 89mg | Fiber: 3g | PCF Ratio: 65-18-17 | Exchange Approx.: 1 Starch, ½ Fruit

INGREDIENTS | SERVES 6

2 large whole eggs

1 large egg white

½ cup skim milk

½ cup all-purpose flour

1 tablespoon granulated sugar

⅛ teaspoon sea salt

2 cups of fresh berries such as raspberries, blackberries, boysenberries, blueberries, strawberries, or a combination

1 tablespoon powdered sugar

Syrup Substitutes

Spreading 2 teaspoons of your favorite Smucker's Low Sugar jam or jelly on a waffle or pancake not only gives you a sweet topping, it can be one of your Free Exchange List choices for the day.

1. Preheat oven to 450°F. Treat 10" ovenproof skillet or deep pie pan with nonstick spray. Once oven is heated, place pan in oven for a few minutes to get hot.

2. Add eggs and egg white to medium bowl; beat until mixed. Whisk in milk. Slowly whisk in flour, sugar, and salt.

3. Remove preheated pan from oven; pour batter into it. Bake for 15 minutes; reduce heat to 350°F and bake for an additional 10 minutes, or until batter is puffed and brown. Remove from oven and slide onto serving plate. Cover with fruit and sift powdered sugar over top. Cut into 6 equal wedges and serve.

Sweet Potato Pancakes

PER SERVING: Calories: 168 | Protein: 6g | Carbohydrates: 287g | Fat: 7g | Saturated Fat: 1g
Cholesterol: 0mg | Sodium: 139mg | Fiber: 3g | PCF Ratio: 13-49-37 | Exchange Approx.: 1 Starch, 1½ Fats

INGREDIENTS | SERVES 4

1½ cups sweet potatoes, cooked
¼ cup onions, grated
1 egg
3 tablespoons whole-wheat pastry flour
½ teaspoon cinnamon
½ teaspoon baking powder
½ cup egg whites
2 tablespoons canola oil

1. Scrub 2 medium sweet potatoes; pierce skins with fork and microwave on high for 4–5 minutes. When sweet potatoes have cooled enough to handle, scoop sweet potato out of skins; lightly mash with fork.

2. In medium bowl, mix together sweet potatoes, grated onion, and egg. Add in flour, cinnamon, and baking powder.

3. In separate small bowl, beat egg whites until rounded peaks are formed. Gently fold egg whites into potato mixture.

4. Heat oil in skillet (nonstick preferably) until hot. Spoon batter onto skillet to form pancakes approximately 4" in diameter. Brown on both sides.

5. Serve hot with unsweetened applesauce.

Egg Clouds on Toast

PER SERVING: Calories: 57 | Protein: 4g | Carbohydrates: 9g | Fat: 1g | Saturated Fat: 0g | Cholesterol: 0mg
Sodium: 101mg | Fiber: 0g | PCF Ratio: 30-63-7 | Exchange Approx.: ½ Very-Lean Fat Meat, ½ Starch

INGREDIENTS | SERVES 1

2 egg whites

½ teaspoon sugar

1 cup water

1 tablespoon frozen apple juice concentrate

1 slice reduced-calorie oat-bran bread, lightly toasted

Tip

Additional serving suggestions: Spread 1 teaspoon of low-sugar or all-fruit spread on toast (½ Fruit Exchange) before ladling on the "clouds." For cinnamon French-style toast, sprinkle ¼ teaspoon cinnamon and ½ teaspoon powdered sugar (less than 10 calories) over top of the clouds.

1. In copper bowl, beat egg whites until thickened. Add sugar; continue to beat until stiff peaks form.

2. In small saucepan, heat water and apple juice over medium heat until it just begins to boil; reduce heat and allow mixture to simmer. Drop egg whites by teaspoonful into simmering water. Simmer for 3 minutes; turn over and simmer for an additional 3 minutes.

3. Ladle "clouds" over bread and serve immediately.

Quinoa Berry Breakfast

PER SERVING: Calories: 228 | Protein: 7g | Carbohydrates: 41g | Fat: 5g | Saturated Fat: 0g | Cholesterol: 0mg
Sodium: 2mg | Fiber: 5g | PCF Ratio: 12-69-19 | Exchange Approx.: 2 Starches, 1 Fruit, 1 Very-Lean Meat, 4 Fats

INGREDIENTS | SERVES 4

1 cup quinoa

2 cups water

¼ cup walnuts

1 teaspoon cinnamon

2 cups berries

Single Serving Quick Tip

Use this basic recipe to make 4 servings at
once. Refrigerated any leftover portions;
microwave 1 to 1½ minutes on high for single portions as needed. Use cooked quinoa
within 3 days. Try other berries, nuts, or
spices such as ginger or nutmeg to vary
this nutritious breakfast cereal.

1. Rinse quinoa in fine-mesh sieve before cooking. Place
   quinoa, water, walnuts, and cinnamon in 1½ quart
   saucepan; bring to a boil. Reduce heat to low; cover
   and cook for 15 minutes, or until all water has been
   absorbed.

2. Add berries and serve with milk, soy milk, or
   sweetener if desired.

CHAPTER 5

Meats

Pork Lo Mein

PER SERVING: Calories: 266 | Protein: 23g | Carbohydrates: 25g | Fat: 8g | Saturated Fat: 2g | Cholesterol: 50mg
Sodium: 386mg | Fiber: 5g | PCF Ratio: 35-38-27 | Exchange Approx.: 2½ Lean Meats, 1 Starch, 1 Vegetable

INGREDIENTS | SERVES 4

1½ tablespoons reduced-sodium soy sauce
1 teaspoon fresh ginger, grated
1 tablespoon rice vinegar
¼ teaspoon turmeric
¾ pound lean pork loin, cut into 1" cubes
½ cup green onion, sliced
2 teaspoons garlic, minced
2 cups cabbage, shredded
1 cup snap peas, cut into 1" pieces
½ tablespoon canola oil
¼ teaspoon crushed red pepper
2 cups whole-grain spaghetti, cooked
1 teaspoon sesame oil
1 teaspoon sesame seeds

1. Combine soy sauce, ginger, rice vinegar, and turmeric in bowl. Mix in cubed pork; set aside.

2. Cut up onion, garlic, cabbage, and snap peas before starting stir-fry.

3. In large skillet or wok, heat oil and sauté onion and garlic. Add meat; cook quickly until meat and onions are slightly browned.

4. Add in cabbage and snap peas; continue to stir-fry for another 3–4 minutes. Sprinkle in crushed red pepper.

5. When vegetables are crisp-tender, add cooked pasta, sesame oil, and sesame seeds. Toss lightly and serve.

Slow-Cooker Pork with Plum Sauce

PER SERVING, with Bragg's Liquid Aminos: Calories: 125 | Protein: 13g | Carbohydrates: 11g | Fat: 3g
Saturated Fat: 1g | Cholesterol: 36mg | Sodium: 148mg | Fiber: 0g | PCF Ratio: 42-37-21
Exchange Approx.: 2 Lean Meats, ½ Fruit

INGREDIENTS | SERVES 4

½ pound (8 ounces) cooked shredded pork
1 clove garlic, crushed
½ teaspoon grated fresh ginger
⅛ cup apple juice
¼ teaspoon dry mustard
2 teaspoons Bragg's Liquid Aminos or soy sauce
⅛ teaspoon dried thyme
⅛ cup plum jam
½ teaspoon cornstarch

1. In nonstick skillet treated with nonstick spray, stir-fry pork, garlic, and ginger for approximately 2 minutes.

2. In small bowl or measuring cup, combine remaining ingredients to make a slurry; pour over the heated pork, mixing well. Cook over low to medium heat until mixture thickens and juice is absorbed into pork, approximately 15 minutes.

Slow-Cooked Venison

PER SERVING: Calories: 90 | Protein: 18g | Carbohydrates: 0g | Fat: 2g | Saturated Fat: 1g
Cholesterol: 64mg | Sodium: 31mg | Fiber: 0g | PCF Ratio: 81-0-19 | Exchange Approx.: 2 Very-Lean Meats

INGREDIENTS	YIELDS ABOUT 1 POUND; SERVING SIZE: 2 OUNCES

1-pound venison roast
1–2 tablespoons cider vinegar

1. Put venison in ceramic-lined slow cooker; add enough water to cover. Add vinegar; set on high. Once mixture begins to boil, reduce temperature to low. Allow meat to simmer for 8 or more hours.

2. Drain resulting broth from meat and discard. Remove any remaining fat from meat and discard. Weigh meat and separate into servings. Meat will keep for 1–2 days in refrigerator, or freeze portions for later use.

Slow-Cooker Venison Barbecue

PER SERVING: Calories: 117 | Protein: 17g | Carbohydrates: 5g | Fat: 2g | Saturated Fat: 1g | Cholesterol: 63mg
Sodium: 185mg | Fiber: .04g | PCF Ratio: 65-20-16 | Exchange Approx.: 2 Very-Lean Meats, 1 Free Condiment

INGREDIENTS	SERVES 12

1½ pounds (24 ounces) Slow-Cooked Venison (recipe above)
1 cup water
½ cup dry white wine
½ cup Brooks Tangy Catsup
1 tablespoon red wine vinegar
1 tablespoon stone-ground mustard
1 tablespoon dried onion flakes
⅛ cup (2 tablespoons) Worcestershire sauce (store bought or made with recipe on page 192)
1 teaspoon dried minced garlic
1 teaspoon cracked black pepper
1 tablespoon brown sugar

Add cooked venison to slow cooker. Mix remaining ingredients together; pour over venison. Add additional water, if necessary, to completely cover meat. Set slow cooker on high until mixture begins to boil. Reduce heat to low and simmer for 2 or more hours. Adjust seasonings, if necessary.

Game Over

Instead of using the slow-cooker method to remove any gamy flavor from game meats, soak it in milk or tomato juice overnight. Drain the meat, and discard the soaking liquid.

Beef Broth: Easy Slow-Cooker Method

PER SERVING: Calories: 58 | Protein: 9g | Carbohydrates: 0g | Fat: 2g | Saturated Fat: 1g
Cholesterol: 27mg | Sodium: 14mg | Fiber: 0g | PCF Ratio: 65-0-35 | Exchange Approx.: 1 Lean Meat

INGREDIENTS | YIELDS ABOUT 3 CUPS BROTH; SERVING SIZE: ½ CUP

1 pound lean round steak
1 onion, chopped
2 carrots, peeled and chopped
2 celery stalks and leaves, chopped
1 bay leaf
4 sprigs parsley
6 black peppercorns
¼ cup dry white wine
4½ cups water

Trade Secrets

Some chefs swear that a hearty beef broth requires oven-roasted bones. Place bones on a roasting tray and bake in 425°F oven for 30–60 minutes. Blot fat from bones before adding to rest of broth ingredients. You may need to reduce the amount of water in your slow cooker, which will produce a more concentrated broth.

1. Cut beef into several pieces; add to slow cooker with all other ingredients. Use high setting until mixture reaches a boil, then reduce heat to low. Allow to simmer, covered, overnight, or up to 16 hours.

2. Remove beef and drain on paper towels to absorb any fat. Strain broth, discarding meat and vegetables. (You don't want to eat vegetables cooked directly with the beef because they will have absorbed too much of the residue fat.) Put broth in a covered container and refrigerate for several hours or overnight; this allows time for fat to congeal on top of broth. Remove hardened fat and discard. (When you remove fat from broth, the Exchange Approximation for it will be a Free Exchange.) Broth will keep in refrigerator for a few days. Freeze any you won't use within that time.

Stovetop Grilled Beef Loin

PER SERVING: Calories: 105 | Protein: 15g | Carbohydrates: 1g | Fat: 4g | Saturated Fat: 1g
Cholesterol: 2mg | Sodium: 27mg | Fiber: 0g | PCF Ratio: 58-5-37 | Exchange Approx.: 2½ Lean Meats

INGREDIENTS | YIELDS 1 (5-OUNCE) LOIN; SERVING SIZE: 2½ OUNCES

1 lean beef tenderloin fillet, no more than 1" thick

½ teaspoon paprika

1½ teaspoons garlic powder

⅛ teaspoon cracked black pepper

¼ teaspoon onion powder

Pinch to ⅛ teaspoon cayenne pepper (according to taste)

⅛ teaspoon dried oregano

⅛ teaspoon dried thyme

½ teaspoon brown sugar

½ teaspoon olive oil

Weights and Measures: Before and After

Exchanges are based on cooking weight of meats; however, in the case of lean pork loin trimmed of all fat, very little weight is lost during the cooking process. Therefore, amounts given for raw pork loin in recipes equal cooked weights. If you find your cooking method causes more variation in weight, adjust accordingly.

1. Remove loin from refrigerator 30 minutes before preparing it to allow it to come to room temperature. Pat meat dry with paper towels.

2. Mix together all dry ingredients. Rub ¼ teaspoon of olive oil on each side of the fillet. (The olive oil is used in this recipe to help the "rub" adhere to the meat and to aid in the caramelization process.) Divide seasoning mixture; rub into each oiled side.

3. Heat a grill pan on high for 1–2 minutes, until the pan is sizzling hot. Place beef fillet in pan, reduce heat to medium-high, and cook 3 minutes. Use tongs to turn fillet. (Be careful not to pierce meat.) Cook for another 2 minutes for medium or 3 minutes for well-done.

4. Remove from heat and let the meat rest in pan for at least 5 minutes, allowing juices to redistribute throughout meat and complete cooking process, which makes for a juicier fillet.

The Ultimate Grilled Cheeseburger Sandwich

PER SERVING: Calories: 262 | Protein: 17g | Carbohydrates: 15g | Fat: 15g | Saturated Fat: 5g | Cholesterol: 60mg
Sodium: 252mg | Fiber: 1.22g | PCF Ratio: 26-24-50 | Exchange Approx.: 2 Lean Meats, 1 Fat, 1 Starch

INGREDIENTS | SERVES 4

1 tablespoon olive oil

1 teaspoon butter

2 thick slices of 7-Grain Bread (page 203)

1 ounce Cheddar cheese

½ pound (8 ounces) ground round

1 teaspoon Worcestershire sauce, or to taste

Fresh minced garlic, to taste

Balsamic vinegar, to taste

Toppings of your choice such as stoneground mustard, mayonnaise, etc.

The Olive Oil Factor

Once you've used an olive oil and butter mixture to butter the bread for a toasted or grilled sandwich, you'll never want to use just plain butter again! Olive oil helps make the bread crunchier and imparts a subtle taste difference to the sandwiches.

1. Preheat indoor grill. Combine olive oil and butter; use ½ to butter 1 side of each slice of bread. Place Cheddar cheese on unbuttered side of 1 slice of bread; top with other slice, buttered-side up.

2. Combine ground round with Worcestershire sauce, garlic, and balsamic vinegar, if using. Shape ground round into large, rectangular patty, a little larger than slice of bread. Grill patty and then cheese sandwich. (If you are using a large indoor grill, position hamburger at lower end, near area where fat drains; grill cheese sandwich at higher end.)

3. Once cheese sandwich is done, separate slices of bread, being careful not to burn yourself on cheese. Top 1 slice with hamburger and add your choice of condiments and fixin's.

Southwest Black Bean Burgers

PER SERVING: Calories: 230 | Protein: 20g | Carbohydrates: 10g | Fat: 12g | Saturated Fat: 4g | Cholesterol: 55mg
Sodium: 102mg | Fiber: 4g | PCF Ratio: 36-18-46 | Exchange Approx.: 2½ Lean Meats, ½ Starch, 1 Fat

INGREDIENTS | SERVES 5

1 cup black beans, cooked

¼ cup onion, chopped

1 teaspoon chili powder

1 teaspoon ground cumin

1 tablespoon fresh parsley, minced

1 tablespoon fresh cilantro, minced

½ teaspoon salt (optional)

¾ pound lean ground beef

Swapping Fresh Herbs for Dried

If you do not have fresh herbs such as parsley or cilantro available, 1 teaspoon dried can be used in place of 1 tablespoon fresh.

1. Place beans, onion, chili powder, cumin, parsley, cilantro, and salt in food processor. Combine ingredients using pulse setting until beans are partially puréed and all ingredients are mixed. (If using canned beans, drain and rinse first.)

2. In a separate bowl, combine ground beef and bean mixture. Shape into 5 patties.

3. Meat mixture is quite soft after mixing and should be chilled or partially frozen prior to cooking. Grill or broil on oiled surface.

Italian Sausage

PER SERVING, without salt: Calories: 135 | Protein: 15g | Carbohydrates: 0g | Fat: 8g | Saturated Fat: 3g
Cholesterol: 45mg | Sodium: 27mg | Fiber: 0g | PCF Ratio: 47-0-53 | Exchange Approx.: 1 Medium-Fat Meat

INGREDIENTS | YIELDS ABOUT 2 POUNDS (32 OUNCES); SERVING SIZE: 2 OUNCES

2 pounds (32 ounces) pork shoulder

1 teaspoon ground black pepper

1 teaspoon dried parsley

1 teaspoon Italian-style seasoning

1 teaspoon garlic powder

¾ teaspoon crushed anise seeds

⅛ teaspoon crushed red pepper flakes

½ teaspoon paprika

½ teaspoon instant minced onion flakes

1 teaspoon kosher or sea salt (optional)

1. Remove all fat from meat; cut the meat into cubes. Put in food processor; grind to desired consistency.

2. Add remaining ingredients; mix until well blended. You can put sausage mixture in casings, but it works equally well broiled or grilled as patties.

Simple (and Smart!) Substitutions

Game meats—buffalo, venison, elk, moose—are low in fat, as are ground chicken or turkey. Substitute one of these for pork in any of the sausage recipes in this chapter.

Italian Sweet Fennel Sausage

PER SERVING, without salt: Calories: 139 | Protein: 15g | Carbohydrates: 1g | Fat: 8g | Saturated Fat: 3g
Cholesterol: 45mg | Sodium: 27mg | Fiber: 0g | PCF Ratio: 46-3-51 | Exchange Approx.: 1 Medium-Fat Meat

INGREDIENTS | YIELDS ABOUT 2 POUNDS (32 OUNCES); SERVING SIZE: 2 OUNCES

2 pounds (32 ounces) pork butt

½ teaspoon black pepper

2½ teaspoons crushed garlic

1 tablespoon sugar

1 teaspoon kosher or sea salt (optional)

1. Toast fennel seeds and cayenne pepper in nonstick skillet over medium heat, stirring constantly, until seeds just begin to darken, about 2 minutes. Set aside.

2. Remove all fat from meat; cut the meat into cubes. Put in food processor; grind to desired consistency. Add remaining ingredients; mix until well blended. You can put sausage mixture in casings, but it works equally well broiled or grilled as patties.

Better the Second Day

Ideally, sausage is made the night before and refrigerated to allow the flavors to merge. Leftover sausage can be frozen for up to 3 months.

Mock Chorizo 1

PER SERVING, without salt: Calories: 137 | Protein: 15g | Carbohydrates: 1g | Fat: 8g | Saturated Fat: 3g
Cholesterol: 45mg | Sodium: 27mg | Fiber: 0g | PCF Ratio: 47-1-52 | Exchange Approx.: 1 Medium-Fat Meat

INGREDIENTS | YIELDS ABOUT 2 POUNDS (32 OUNCES); SERVING SIZE: 2 OUNCES

2 pounds (32 ounces) lean pork

4 tablespoons chili powder

¼ teaspoon ground cloves

2 tablespoons paprika

2½ teaspoons crushed fresh garlic

1 teaspoon crushed dried oregano

3½ tablespoons cider vinegar

1 teaspoon kosher or sea salt (optional)

1. Remove all fat from meat; cut the meat into cubes. Put in food processor; grind to desired consistency. Add remaining ingredients; mix until well blended.

2. Tradition calls for aging this sausage in an airtight container in the refrigerator for 4 days before cooking. Leftover sausage can be stored in the freezer up to 3 months.

Break from Tradition

Traditionally, chorizo is very high in fat. The chorizo recipes in this chapter are lower-fat alternatives. They make excellent replacements for adding flavor to recipes that call for bacon. In fact, 1 or 2 ounces of chorizo can replace an entire pound of bacon in cabbage, bean, or potato soup.

Mock Chorizo 2

PER SERVING, without salt: Calories: 140 | Protein: 16g | Carbohydrates: 1g | Fat: 8g | Saturated Fat: 3g | Cholesterol: 45mg
Sodium: 27mg | Fiber: 0g | PCF Ratio: 46-2-52 | Exchange Approx.: 1 Medium-Fat Meat

INGREDIENTS | YIELDS ABOUT 1 POUND (16 OUNCES); SERVING SIZE: 2 OUNCES

1 pound (16 ounces) lean pork

2 tablespoons white wine vinegar

1 tablespoon dry sherry

2 teaspoons paprika

2 teaspoons chili powder

½ teaspoon dried oregano

¼ teaspoon ground cumin

½ teaspoon freshly ground black pepper

⅛ teaspoon ground cinnamon

⅛ teaspoon ground cloves

Pinch of ground coriander

Pinch of ground ginger

2 cloves garlic, crushed

Kosher or sea salt, to taste (optional)

Tip

For chorizo stir-fry, consider decreasing the chili powder, adding some soy sauce or Bragg's Liquid Aminos, and increasing the garlic and ginger.

1. Remove all fat from meat; cut the meat into cubes. Put in food processor; grind to desired consistency. Add remaining ingredients; mix until well blended.

2. Age sausage in an airtight container in the refrigerator for 4 days. Leftover sausage can be stored in the freezer up to 3 months.

Kousa (Squash Stuffed with Lamb and Rice)

PER SERVING: Calories: 430 | Protein: 27g | Carbohydrates: 36g | Fat: 20g | Saturated Fat: 7g | Cholesterol: 82mg
Sodium: 692mg | Fiber: 5g | PCF Ratio: 25-33-42 | Exchange Approx.: 3 Lean Meats, 1 Starch, 3 Vegetables, 3 Fats

INGREDIENTS | SERVES 4

3 cups tomatoes, chopped

1 cup onion, chopped

2 cups water

½ teaspoon salt

⅛ teaspoon fresh ground pepper

2 tablespoons fresh mint, minced

4 small zucchini squash (7"–8" long)

¾ pound very lean ground lamb

½ cup rice

2 tablespoons pine nuts

½ teaspoon salt

⅛ teaspoon allspice

⅛ teaspoon fresh ground pepper

Summer Harvest

Kousa (stuffed squash) is a traditional Lebanese dish that uses a pale green summer squash very similar to zucchini. This squash is not always easy to find, but zucchini is very abundant and works quite well. If you have a large garden crop of zucchini: Pick them small, hollow out the squash, blanch in boiling water for 2 minutes, then freeze. You'll have squash ready to stuff all year long.

1. Prepare tomato sauce first: Combine tomatoes, onion, water, salt, pepper, and fresh mint in a large pot. Bring to a boil; reduce heat and simmer 30 minutes.

2. Scrub squash and dry with paper towels. Remove stem ends of each squash and carefully core center, leaving about ¼" of shell.

3. Make stuffing: thoroughly mix ground lamb, rice, pine nuts, salt, allspice, and pepper.

4. Spoon stuffing into each squash, tapping bottom end of squash to get stuffing down. Fill each squash to top; stuffing should be loosely packed to allow rice to expand while cooking.

5. Place squash in tomato sauce, lying them on their sides. Bring sauce to a slow boil; cover and cook over low heat for 45–60 minutes, or until squash is tender and rice has cooked. Serve squash with tomato sauce spooned over top.

Baked Stuffed Kibbeh

**PER SERVING: Calories: 226 | Protein: 18g | Carbohydrates: 13g | Fat: 12g | Saturated Fat: 4g | Cholesterol: 62mg
Sodium: 343mg | Fiber: 3g | PCF Ratio: 32-22-46 | Exchange Approx.: 1 Starch, 2 Lean Meats, 2 Fats**

INGREDIENTS | SERVES 8

Cooking spray
¾ cup bulgur wheat, fine grind
2 cups boiling water
1 pound lean ground lamb
1 cup onion, grated
1 teaspoon salt
¼ teaspoon pepper
Small bowl ice water
1½ tablespoons butter
¼ cup pine nuts
¼ teaspoon cinnamon
¼ teaspoon allspice
1½ tablespoons butter

Making Lean Ground Lamb

Unless you have a butcher, very lean ground lamb is difficult to find. Make it yourself using chunks of meat trimmed from a leg of lamb. Be sure to remove all visible fat from the lamb and grind twice using a medium or fine grinder blade. Removing all visible fat prevents lamb from having a strong "mutton" taste.

1. Spray 9" × 9" baking dish with cooking spray.

2. Put bulgur wheat in small bowl. Cover with boiling water and allow wheat to absorb liquid, approximately 15–20 minutes.

3. Line colander with small piece of cheesecloth. Drop bulgur wheat into cloth; drain and squeeze as much liquid out of wheat as possible.

4. On large cutting board, combine lamb, ½ grated onions, wheat, salt, and pepper; mix with hands, kneading together all ingredients.

5. Divide meat mixture in ½. Place ½ in bottom of baking dish by dipping hands into ice water to spread meat mixture smoothly over bottom of dish. Cover bottom of dish completely.

6. In a small pan, melt 1½ tablespoons of butter; sauté remaining onions, pine nuts, cinnamon, and allspice until onions are soft.

7. Spread onion and pine nut mixture evenly over first layer of meat in baking dish. Take remaining ½ of meat mixture and spread smoothly on top, using procedure in Step 5.

8. Score top in diamond shapes with a knife dipped in cold water. Melt remaining 1½ tablespoons of butter; drizzle over top of meat. Bake at 350°F for approximately 40–45 minutes, or until golden brown.

Slow-Cooker Beef Braciole

PER SERVING: Calories: 367 | Protein: 29g | Carbohydrates: 293g | Fat: 16g | Saturated Fat: 5g
Cholesterol: 69mg | Sodium: 162mg | Fiber: 5g | PCF Ratio: 32-29-39 | Exchange Approx.: 3½
Very-Lean Meats, 2½ Fats, 3 Vegetables, 1 Starch

INGREDIENTS | SERVES 4

4 cups tomato sauce

1 tablespoon olive oil

¼ cup onion, finely chopped

1 teaspoon garlic, finely chopped

¼ cup carrots, finely chopped

¼ cup celery, finely chopped

2 slices whole-wheat bread, cubed

1 egg, lightly beaten

1 pound thinly sliced round beef, cut into 4 pieces

1. Prepare tomato sauce in slow cooker (see page 139 or use your own sauce recipe) in advance and maintain at medium heat.

2. Heat olive oil in large nonstick skillet; sauté onions, garlic, carrots, and celery until softened. Remove from heat.

3. Add cubed bread and egg to sautéed vegetables; mix well.

4. Pound each piece of beef on both sides to flatten and tenderize. Each slice of meat should be about ¼" thick. Place approximately ½ cup of bread and vegetable stuffing down center of each meat slice and press in place. Starting at one end, roll meat up like a jelly roll; secure with 6" wooden skewer.

5. Place meat rolls in tomato sauce. Set slow cooker on low to medium setting; cook for at least 4 hours. (On low setting, the meat rolls can be left in slow cooker for 6–8 hours.) Remove wooden skewers before serving.

Soy and Ginger Flank Steak

PER SERVING: Calories: 304 | Protein: 29g | Carbohydrates: 1g | Fat: 19g | Saturated Fat: 7g | Cholesterol: 95mg
Sodium: 213mg | Fiber: 0g | PCF Ratio: 40-2-58 | Exchange Approx.: 4 Lean Meats, 1½ Fats

INGREDIENTS | SERVES 4

1 pound lean London broil
1 tablespoon fresh ginger, minced
2 teaspoons fresh garlic, minced
1 tablespoon reduced-sodium soy sauce
3 tablespoons dry red wine
¼ teaspoon pepper
½ tablespoon olive oil

Slicing Meats Against the Grain

Certain cuts of meat such as flank steak, brisket, and London broil have a distinct grain (or line) of fibers running through them. If you slice with the grain, meat will seem tough and difficult to chew. These cuts of meat should always be thinly sliced across (or against) the grain so fibers are cut through so meats remain tender and easy to chew.

1. Marinate meat at least 3–4 hours in advance. Place meat, ginger, garlic, soy sauce, red wine, pepper, and olive oil in shallow baking dish. Coat meat with marinade on both sides.

2. Cover and refrigerate meat in marinade, turning meat once or twice during marinating so all marinade soaks into both sides of meat.

3. Lightly oil barbecue grill and preheat. Place flank steak on grill. Grill steak, turning once, until done to your preference. Medium-rare will take approximately 12–15 minutes. Slice meat diagonally and against grain into thin slices.

Pork Roast with Caramelized Onions and Apples

PER SERVING: Calories: 373 | Protein: 31g | Carbohydrates: 8g | Fat: 23g | Saturated Fat: 9g | Cholesterol: 96mg
Sodium: 156mg | Fiber: 1g | PCF Ratio: 34-9-57 | Exchange Approx.: 1 Vegetable, 4 Lean Meats, 2 Fats

INGREDIENTS | SERVES 6

2 pounds lean pork loin roast
Fresh ground pepper
½ tablespoon olive oil
½ tablespoon butter
2 cups onion, chopped
1 tablespoon Marsala wine
⅓ cup low-sodium chicken broth
1 apple, peeled and chopped

1. Preheat oven to 375°F. Season pork loin with pepper. Heat olive oil in a large skillet; sear to brown all sides.

2. Transfer roast to 9" × 13" glass baking dish; place in oven for approximately 1 hour and 15 minutes.

3. While pork is roasting, prepare onions: In large nonstick skillet, melt butter and add onions. Sauté onions until soft; add wine, chicken broth, and apple. Continue cooking on low heat until onions are soft, brown in color, and have caramelized.

4. When roast has reached an internal temperature of 130°F, spoon onions over top; place a loose foil tent over roast.

5. Remove roast from oven when an internal temperature of 145°F has been reached. (Temperature of roast will continue to rise as meat rests.) Keep roast loosely covered with foil and allow to stand for 10–15 minutes before slicing.

Sweet and Sour Pork Skillet

PER SERVING: Calories: 198 | Protein: 26g | Carbohydrates: 12g | Fat: 5g | Saturated Fat: 2g
Cholesterol: 67mg | Sodium: 164mg | Fiber: 3g | PCF Ratio: 47-30-25 | Exchange Approx.: 3½
Very-Lean Meats, 1½ Vegetables, ½ Other Carbohydrate, ½ Fat

INGREDIENTS | SERVES 4

12 ounces lean pork tenderloin

1 tablespoon honey

2 tablespoons rice vinegar or white vinegar

2 teaspoons soy sauce

½ teaspoon grated ginger

½ cup onions, chopped

½ cup carrots, julienne cut

2 cups cauliflower florets

¼ teaspoon Chinese five spice powder

Aromatic Five Spice Powder

Chinese five spice powder is a blend of cinnamon, anise, fennel (or star anise), ginger, and clove. Five spice powder is an essential base seasoning for many Chinese dishes. A little of this aromatic mix goes a long way, giving dishes a hint of sweet, savory, and sour.

1. Cut pork into 1" strips. In medium bowl, combine pork, honey, vinegar, soy sauce, and ginger. Coat pork strips with mixture; allow to marinate for at least 15 minutes.

2. Heat large nonstick skillet or wok. Add pork strips and onion; quickly stir-fry over high heat for 2–3 minutes. Reserve any leftover marinade to add with vegetables.

3. Add carrots, cauliflower, and marinade. Toss all ingredients and continue to stir-fry, allowing marinade to coat all vegetables. Cook over high heat for an additional 3–4 minutes, or until vegetables are crisp-tender.

4. Add five spice powder and combine just before serving.

Fruited Pork Loin Roast Casserole

PER SERVING: Calories: 170 | Protein: 7g | Carbohydrates: 27g | Fat: 4g | Saturated Fat: 1g | Cholesterol: 19mg
Sodium: 32mg | Fiber: 3g | PCF Ratio: 17-63-20 | Exchange Approx.: 1 Lean Meat, 1 Fruit, 1 Starch

INGREDIENTS | SERVES 4

4 small Yukon Gold potatoes, peeled and sliced

2 (2-ounce) pieces trimmed boneless pork loin, pounded flat

1 apple, peeled, cored, and sliced

4 apricot halves

1 tablespoon chopped red onion or shallot

⅛ cup apple cider or apple juice

Optional seasonings, to taste:

   Olive oil

   Parmesan cheese

   Salt and freshly ground pepper

1. Preheat oven to 350°F (325°F if using a glass casserole dish); treat casserole dish with nonstick spray.

2. Layer ½ of potato slices across bottom of dish; top with 1 piece of flattened pork loin. Arrange apple slices over top of loin; place apricot halves on top of apple. Sprinkle red onion over apricot and apples. Add second flattened pork loin; layer remaining potatoes atop loin. Drizzle apple cider over top of casserole.

3. Cover and bake for 45 minutes to 1 hour, or until potatoes are tender. Keep casserole covered and let sit for 10 minutes after removing from oven.

Tip

To enhance the flavor of this dish, top with the optional ingredients when it's served. Just be sure to make the appropriate Exchange Approximations adjustments if you do.

White Wine and Lemon Pork Roast

PER SERVING: Calories: 172 | Protein: 18g | Carbohydrates: 2g | Fat: 7g | Saturated Fat: 2g
Cholesterol: 50mg | Sodium: 47mg | Fiber: 0g | PCF Ratio: 53-5-42 | Exchange Approx.: 3 Lean Meats

INGREDIENTS | SERVES 4

1 clove garlic, crushed

½ cup dry white wine

1 tablespoon lemon juice

1 teaspoon olive oil

1 tablespoon minced red onion or shallot

¼ teaspoon dried thyme

⅛ teaspoon ground black pepper

12 ounces pork loin roast

1. Make marinade by combining garlic, white wine, lemon juice, olive oil, red onion, thyme, and black pepper in heavy, freezer-style plastic bag. Add roast; marinate in refrigerator 1 hour or overnight, according to taste. (Note: Pork loin is already tender, so you're marinating the meat to impart the flavors only.)

2. Preheat oven to 350°F. Remove meat from marinade; put on nonstick spray–treated rack in roasting pan. Roast for 20–30 minutes, or until meat thermometer reads 150°F to 170°F, depending on how well done you prefer it.

Marmalade Marinade

Combine 1 teaspoon Dijon or stone-ground mustard, 1 tablespoon Smucker's Low-Sugar Orange Marmalade, 1 clove crushed garlic, and ¼ teaspoon dried thyme leaves. Marinate and prepare a ½-pound (8-ounce) pork loin as you would the White Wine and Lemon Pork Loin Roast. The Nutritional Analysis for a 2-ounce serving is: Calories: 89.52; Protein: 126g; Carbohydrate: 1.90g; Fat: 26g; Saturated Fat: 1.11g; Cholesterol: 345mg; Sodium: 466mg; Fiber: 0.09g; PCF Ratio: 57-9-34; Exchange Approximations: 2 Lean Meats.

Pecan-Crusted Roast Pork Loin

PER SERVING: Calories: 209 | Protein: 24g | Carbohydrates: 2g | Fat: 11g | Saturated Fat: 2g | Cholesterol: 67mg
Sodium: 47mg | Fiber: 1g | PCF Ratio: 47-4-49 | Exchange Approx.: 3½ Very-Lean Meats, 2 Fats

INGREDIENTS | SERVES 4

1 teaspoon olive oil

1 clove garlic, crushed

1 teaspoon brown sugar

Thyme, sage, and pepper, to taste (optional)

¼ cup chopped or ground pecans

12 ounces boneless pork loin roast

Create a Celery Roasting Rack

If you prefer to bake a loin roast in a casserole alongside potatoes and carrots, elevate the roast on 2 or 3 stalks of celery. The celery will absorb any fat that drains from the meat so that it's not absorbed by the other vegetables. After cooking, discard the celery.

1. Put olive oil, crushed garlic, brown sugar, and seasonings (if using) in a heavy, freezer-style plastic bag. Work bag until ingredients are mixed. Add roast; turn in bag to coat. Marinate in refrigerator for several hours or overnight.

2. Preheat oven to 400°F. Roll pork loin in chopped pecans; place in roasting pan. Make a tent of aluminum foil; arrange over pork loin, covering nuts completely so they won't char. Roast for 10 minutes, then lower heat to 350°F. Continue to roast for another 8–15 minutes, or until meat thermometer reads 150°F to 170°F, depending on how well done you prefer it.

Balsamic Venison Pot Roast

PER SERVING: Calories: 188 | Protein: 28g | Carbohydrates: 6g | Fat: 6g | Saturated Fat: 2g | Cholesterol: 96mg
Sodium: 75mg | Fiber: 1g | PCF Ratio: 60-13-28 | Exchange Approx.: 4 Very Lean Meats, ½ Fat

INGREDIENTS | SERVES 8

2½ tablespoons all-purpose flour

2 teaspoons paprika

2-pound venison roast

1½ tablespoons olive oil

14 ounces low-sodium beef broth

½ cup onion, chopped

2 tablespoons dried onion flakes

⅓ cup balsamic vinegar

⅛ teaspoon Worcestershire sauce

1 teaspoon sugar

1. Mix flour and paprika together; dredge venison in flour mixture and completely coat with flour.

2. Heat oil in Dutch oven or deep skillet; brown roast on all sides.

3. Add beef broth, onion, onion flakes, balsamic vinegar, Worcestershire sauce, and sugar. Bring to a quick boil; reduce heat to low.

4. Cover and cook over low heat for 2–3 hours, or until venison is tender and cuts easily. Serve with whole-grain noodles.

Recipe Adaptation

This recipe also works well cooked in a slow cooker for 6–8 hours, until tender. Slow cookers with a ceramic interior maintain low temperatures better than those with a metal cooking surface.

Venison Pepper Steak

PER SERVING: Calories: 237 | Protein: 26g | Carbohydrates: 12g | Fat: 9g | Saturated Fat: 3g | Cholesterol: 39mg
Sodium: 344mg | Fiber: 2g | PCF Ratio: 44-20-36 | Exchange Approx.: 3½ Very-Lean Meats, 2 Vegetables, 1½ Fats

INGREDIENTS | SERVES 4

1 pound venison loin
2 tablespoons reduced-sodium soy sauce
1 clove garlic
1½ teaspoons ginger, grated
1 tablespoon canola oil
1 cup onion, thinly sliced
1 cup green or red peppers, cut into ½" strips
½ cup celery, thinly sliced
1 tablespoon cornstarch
1 cup water
1½ cups tomatoes, chopped

1. Cut meat across grain into ¼" strips.

2. Combine soy sauce, garlic, and ginger in bowl. Add sliced meat; mix well and set aside.

3. Heat canola oil in large wok or skillet. Add meat and cook for 2–3 minutes over high heat. Cover, reduce heat, and simmer for 15 minutes.

4. Add onions, peppers, and celery to meat; cover and cook on low heat for another 15 minutes, or until sliced meat is tender.

5. Mix cornstarch with water; add to meat. Cook for 5 minutes, or until sauce thickens slightly. Add tomatoes and heat through.

Whole Grain Additions

Instead of serving white rice, substitute brown rice or quinoa mixed with sautéed vegetables with this dish.

Slow-Cooker Venison and Vegetable Pot Roast

PER SERVING: Calories: 309 | Protein: 27g | Carbohydrates: 28g | Fat: 10g | Saturated Fat: 3g
Cholesterol: 39mg | Sodium: 237mg | Fiber: 4g | PCF Ratio: 35-36-28 | Exchange Approx.:
3½ Very-Lean Meats, 1 Starch, 3 Vegetables, 1½ Fats

INGREDIENTS | SERVES 4

1-pound venison roast

1 tablespoon all-purpose flour

1 tablespoon olive oil

1 tablespoon instant brown gravy mix

1 teaspoon Worcestershire sauce

1 cup onions, chopped

½ pound potatoes, cut into 1" pieces

1 cup carrots, cut into 1" pieces

1 cup celery, chopped

½ cup crushed tomato

½ teaspoon dried thyme leaves

1. Dredge roast in flour. Heat olive oil in large skillet; sear roast until browned on all sides. Put roast in slow cooker.

2. Sprinkle instant gravy mix and Worcestershire sauce over top of roast. Place onions, potatoes, carrots, and celery around roast; spoon crushed tomatoes evenly around vegetables. Sprinkle thyme over meat and vegetables.

3. Cook in slow cooker on low setting for 6–8 hours.

Variation

You can also use ⅓ cup water and 2 tablespoons red wine for the liquid instead of crushed tomatoes.

Venison with Dried Cranberry Vinegar Sauce

PER SERVING, without cornstarch or flour: Calories: 154 | Protein: 17g | Carbohydrates: 4g | Fat: 6g
Saturated Fat: 2g | Cholesterol: 69mg | Sodium: 77mg | Fiber: 0g | PCF Ratio: 49-12-38 | Exchange
Approx.: 3 Very Low-Fat Meats, 1 Fat

INGREDIENTS | SERVES 4

⅛ cup (2 tablespoons) dried cranberries

1 tablespoon sugar

3 tablespoons water

⅛ cup (2 tablespoons) champagne or white wine vinegar

2 teaspoons olive oil

1 tablespoon minced shallots or red onion

1 teaspoon minced garlic

⅛ cup (2 tablespoons) dry red wine

½ cup low-fat, reduced-sodium chicken broth

½ teaspoon cracked black pepper

½ pound (8 ounces) Slow-Cooked Venison (page 55)

1 teaspoon cornstarch or potato flour

2 teaspoons butter

Operate Your Appliances Safely

When puréeing hot mixtures, leave the vent uncovered on your food processor. If using a blender, either remove the vent cover from the lid or leave the lid ajar so the steam can escape.

1. Add cranberries, sugar, water, and champagne to saucepan; bring to a boil. Reduce heat and simmer 5 minutes. Remove from heat and transfer to food processor or blender; process until cranberries are chopped (it isn't necessary to purée because you want some cranberry "chunks" to remain). Set aside.

2. Pour olive oil into a heated nonstick skillet. Add shallots and garlic; sauté for 30 seconds. Deglaze pan with red wine; cook, stirring occasionally, until wine is reduced by half. Add cranberry mixture and chicken broth; bring to a boil. Reduce heat to medium-low; season with pepper, add venison, and simmer for 3 minutes, or until meat is heated through.

3. Thicken sauce using a slurry of cornstarch or potato flour and 1 tablespoon of water; simmer until sauce thickens. You'll need to cook the sauce a bit longer if you use cornstarch in order to remove the starchy taste. Remove from heat; add butter and whisk to incorporate into sauce.

CHAPTER 6

Poultry

Pineapple-Orange Grilled Chicken Breasts

PER SERVING: Calories: 165 | Protein: 27g | Carbohydrates: 10g | Fat: 2g | Saturated Fat: 0g
Cholesterol: 58.40mg | Sodium: 75mg | Fiber: 0g | PCF Ratio: 67-25-9 | Exchange Approx.:
3½ Lean Meats, ½ Fruit

INGREDIENTS | SERVES 4

6 ounces pineapple juice

4 ounces orange juice

¼ cup cider vinegar

1 tablespoon fresh tarragon, chopped

½ tablespoon fresh rosemary

1 pound boneless chicken breast, skinned and cut into 4 pieces

1. Mix marinade in large shallow dish 3–4 hours before grilling: pineapple juice, orange juice, vinegar, tarragon, and rosemary.

2. Add raw chicken breasts to marinade; cover and refrigerate 3–4 hours. Turn pieces of chicken to cover with marinade.

3. Heat grill to medium-high; place chicken on grill. Grill approximately 7–10 minutes on each side, until chicken is cooked through.

Spicy Grilled Turkey Burgers

PER SERVING: Calories: 176 | Protein: 26g | Carbohydrates: 5g | Fat: 5g | Saturated Fat: 2g | Cholesterol: 125mg
Sodium: 155mg | Fiber: 0g | PCF Ratio: 63-12-25 | Exchange Approx.: 3½ Very-Lean Meats, 1 Fat

INGREDIENTS | SERVES 4

1 pound ground turkey

¼ cup bread crumbs

1 tablespoon Cajun-blend seasoning (Appendix C) or commercial salt-free blend

1 egg

1 tablespoon fresh cilantro, finely chopped

2 teaspoons jalapeño pepper, minced

Nonstick cooking spray

1. Combine all ingredients well; shape into 4 patties.

2. Spray grill with nonstick cooking spray. Grill burgers approximately 6 minutes on each side, or until cooked through.

Proper Poultry and Meat Handling

Be sure to wash any utensil that comes in contact with raw poultry in hot, soapy water and rinse well. This includes washing any utensil each time it's used to baste grilling, roasting, or baking poultry.

Turkey Kielbasa with Red Beans and Rice

PER SERVING: Calories: 297 | Protein: 15g | Carbohydrates: 41g | Fat: 9g | Saturated Fat: 3g | Cholesterol: 32mg
Sodium: 679mg | Fiber: 7g | PCF Ratio: 19-54-26 | Exchange Approx.: 2 Starches, 1½ Vegetables,
1 Lean Meat, 1 Very-Lean Meat, 3 Fats

INGREDIENTS | SERVES 5

2 cups canned pinto beans, drained and rinsed

2 cups canned diced tomatoes

½ cup water

1 cup onion, diced

2 teaspoons Cajun-blend seasoning (Appendix C)

8 ounces turkey kielbasa sausage, cut into 1" pieces

½ cup brown rice

1½ cups water

1. Combine pinto beans, canned tomatoes, water, onion, Cajun seasoning, and kielbasa in slow cooker; set on low and cook 4–6 hours.

2. In separate saucepan, bring brown rice and 1½ cups water to boil; reduce heat and simmer on low heat 35–40 minutes.

3. Serve beans and sausage over rice.

Herbed Chicken and Brown Rice Dinner

PER SERVING: Calories: 300 | Protein: 33g | Carbohydrates: 26g | Fat: 6g | Saturated Fat: 1g
Cholesterol: 75mg | Sodium: 112mg | Fiber: 0g | PCF Ratio: 45-36-19 | Exchange Approx.: 1½ Starches
2 Very-Lean Meats, 2 Lean Meats

INGREDIENTS | SERVES 4

1 tablespoon canola oil

4 (4-ounce) boneless chicken breast pieces, skin removed

¾ teaspoon garlic powder

¾ teaspoon dried rosemary

1 (10.5-ounce) can low-fat, reduced-sodium chicken broth

⅓ cup water

2 cups uncooked instant brown rice

1. Heat oil in large nonstick skillet on medium-high. Add chicken; sprinkle with ½ of garlic powder and crushed rosemary. Cover, and cook 4 minutes on each side, or until cooked through. Remove chicken from skillet and set aside.

2. Add broth and water to skillet; stir to deglaze pan and bring to a boil. Stir in rice and remaining garlic powder and rosemary. Top with chicken and cover; cook on low heat 5 minutes. Remove from heat and let stand, covered, 5 minutes.

Another Healthy "Fried" Chicken

PER SERVING: Calories: 118 | Protein: 19g | Carbohydrates: 5g | Fat: 2g | Saturated Fat: 1g | Cholesterol: 44mg
Sodium: 91mg | Fiber: 0g | PCF Ratio: 66-18-16 | Exchange Approx.: 2 Very-Lean Meats, ½ Starch

INGREDIENTS | SERVES 4

10 ounces raw boneless, skinless chicken breasts (fat trimmed off)

½ cup nonfat plain yogurt

½ cup bread crumbs

1 teaspoon garlic powder

1 teaspoon paprika

¼ teaspoon dried thyme

Chicken Fat Facts

When faced with the decision of whether to have chicken with or without the skin, consider that ½ pound of skinless chicken breast has 9 grams of fat; ½ pound with the skin on has 38 grams!

1. Preheat oven to 350°F. Prepare baking pan with nonstick cooking spray. Cut chicken breast into 4 equal pieces; marinate in yogurt for several minutes.

2. Mix together bread crumbs, garlic, paprika, and thyme; dredge chicken in crumb mixture. Arrange on prepared pan; bake 20 minutes. To give chicken a deep golden color, place pan under broiler last 5 minutes of cooking. Watch closely to ensure chicken "crust" doesn't burn.

Walnut Chicken with Plum Sauce

PER SERVING: Calories: 159 | Protein: 18g | Carbohydrates: 1g | Fat: 9g | Saturated Fat: 1g | Cholesterol: 44mg
Sodium: 51mg | Fiber: 1g | PCF Ratio: 47-3-51 | Exchange Approx.: 2 Very-Lean Meats, 1½ Fats

INGREDIENTS | SERVES 4

¾ pound (12 ounces) raw boneless, skinless chicken breast

1 teaspoon sherry

1 egg white

2 teaspoons peanut oil

2 drops toasted sesame oil (optional)

⅓ cup ground walnuts

1. Preheat oven to 350°F. Cut chicken into bite-sized pieces; sprinkle with sherry and set aside.

2. In a small bowl, beat egg white and oils until frothy. Fold chicken pieces into egg mixture; roll individually in chopped walnuts.

3. Arrange chicken pieces on baking sheet treated with nonstick cooking spray. Bake 10–15 minutes, or until walnuts are lightly browned and chicken juices run clear. (Walnuts make the fat ratio of this dish high, so serve it with steamed vegetables and rice to bring the ratios into balance.)

Chicken Breasts in Balsamic Vinegar Sauce

PER SERVING: Calories: 200 | Protein: 28g | Carbohydrates: 2g | Fat: 8g | Saturated Fat: 3g | Cholesterol: 73mg
Sodium: 381mg | Fiber: 0g | PCF Ratio: 58-4-38 | Exchange Approx.: 4 Lean Meats, 1½ Fats

INGREDIENTS | SERVES 4

1 pound boneless, skinless chicken breasts, cut into 4 pieces
Pinch salt
¼ teaspoon pepper
1 tablespoon butter
1 tablespoon olive oil
¼ cup red onion, chopped
2 teaspoons garlic, finely chopped
3 tablespoons balsamic vinegar
1½ cups low sodium chicken broth
1 teaspoon oregano

1. Sprinkle chicken with salt and pepper.

2. Heat butter and olive oil in large skillet over medium heat. Add chicken; cook until browned, about 5 minutes each side. Reduce heat and cook 12 minutes. Transfer to platter; cover and keep warm.

3. Add red onions and garlic to skillet; sauté over medium heat 3 minutes, scraping up browned bits. Add balsamic vinegar; bring to a boil. Boil 3 minutes, or until reduced to a glaze, stirring constantly.

4. Add chicken stock; boil until reduced to about ¾ cup liquid. Remove sauce from heat; add chopped oregano. Spoon sauce over chicken and serve immediately.

Turkey Chili

PER SERVING: Calories: 281 | Protein: 26g | Carbohydrates: 38g | Fat: 4g | Saturated Fat: 1g | Cholesterol: 49mg
Sodium: 347mg | Fiber: 11g | PCF Ratio: 35-52-13 | Exchange Approx.: 2 Starches, 2 Vegetables,
3 Very-Lean Meats, 1½ Fats

INGREDIENTS | SERVES 6

1 pound ground turkey
1 cup onions, chopped
½ cup green pepper, chopped
2 teaspoons garlic, finely chopped
2 (28-ounce) cans crushed canned tomatoes
1 cup canned black beans, drained
1 cup canned red kidney beans, drained
3 tablespoons chili powder
1 tablespoon ground cumin
1 teaspoon crushed red pepper
Dash Tabasco

1. Brown ground turkey in large nonstick pot over medium-high heat.

2. Drain off any fat; add chopped onion, green pepper, and garlic. Continue cooking until onion is translucent, about 5 minutes. Add remaining ingredients; bring to a slow boil.

3. Reduce heat, cover, and let simmer at least 2–3 hours before serving.

Chicken Broth: Easy Slow-Cooker Method

PER SERVING: Calories: 67 | Protein: 9g | Carbohydrates: 0g | Fat: 3g | Saturated Fat: 1g | Cholesterol: 24mg
Sodium: 22mg | Fiber: 0g | PCF Ratio: 53-0-47 | Exchange Approx.: ½ Very-Lean Meat, ½ Lean Meat

INGREDIENTS | YIELD ABOUT 4 CUPS; SERVING SIZE: ½ CUP

1 small onion, chopped
2 carrots, peeled and chopped
2 celery stalks and leaves, chopped
1 bay leaf
4 sprigs parsley
6 black peppercorns
¼ cup dry white wine
2 pounds chicken pieces, skin removed
4½ cups water

Reduced Broth

Reducing broth is the act of boiling it to decrease the amount of water so you're left with a richer broth. Boiling nonfat, canned chicken broth won't reduce it as a home-made broth would. The broth from this recipe will be richer than what most recipes call for, so unless you need reduced broth, thin it with water as needed. Assuming you remove the fat from the broth, it will be a Free Exchange.

1. Add all ingredients except water to slow cooker. The chicken pieces and vegetables should be loosely layered and fill no more than ¾ of slow cooker. Add enough water to just cover ingredients; cover slow cooker. Use high setting until mixture almost reaches a boil, then reduce heat to low. Allow to simmer overnight or up to 16 hours, checking occasionally and adding more water, if necessary.

2. Remove chicken pieces and drain on paper towels to absorb any fat. Allow to cool; remove meat from bones. Strain vegetables from broth and discard. (You don't want to eat vegetables cooked directly with chicken because they will have absorbed too much of the residue fat.) Put broth in a covered container; refrigerate for several hours or overnight, allowing fat to congeal on top. Remove hardened fat and discard.

3. To separate broth into small amounts for use when you steam vegetables or potatoes, fill up an ice cube tray with stock. Let freeze, then remove cubes from tray and store in labeled freezer bag. Common ice cube trays allow for ⅛ cup or 2 tablespoons of liquid per section.

Oven-Fried Chicken Thighs

PER SERVING, no oil: Calories: 74 | Protein: 9g | Carbohydrates: 5g | Fat: 2g | Saturated Fat: 1g
Cholesterol: 34mg | Sodium: 331mg | Fiber: 0g | PCF Ratio: 53-26-21 | Exchange Approx.: 2 Very-Lean Meats

INGREDIENTS | SERVES 4

4 chicken thighs, skin removed

1 tablespoon unbleached, white all-purpose flour

1 large egg white

½ teaspoon sea salt

½ teaspoon olive oil (optional; see Comparison Analysis for using olive oil)

1 tablespoon rice flour

1 tablespoon cornmeal

If You Use Oil . . .

Comparison Analysis (with olive oil): Calories: 78.53; Protein: 9.46g; Carbohydrate: 65g; Fat: 27g; Saturated Fat: 0.50g; Cholesterol: 303mg; Sodium: 331.03mg; Fiber: 0.06g; PCF Ratio: 49-24-27; Exchange Approx.: 2 Lean Meats.

1. Preheat oven to 350°F. Rinse and dry chicken thighs. Put white flour on plate. In small, shallow bowl, whip egg white with the sea salt. Add olive oil, if using; mix well. Put rice flour and cornmeal on another plate; mix together. Place rack on baking sheet; spray both with nonstick cooking spray.

2. Roll each chicken thigh in white flour, dip it into egg mixture, and roll in rice flour mixture. Place thighs on rack so they aren't touching. Bake 35–45 minutes, until meat juices run clear.

Buttermilk Ranch Chicken Salad

PER SERVING: Calories: 147 | Protein: 18g | Carbohydrates: 11g | Fat: 4g | Saturated Fat: 1g | Cholesterol: 33mg
Sodium: 184mg | Fiber: 2g | PCF Ratio: 49-29-22 | Exchange Approx.: 2 Very-Lean Meats, ½ Vegetable,
1 Free Vegetable, ½ Skim Milk

INGREDIENTS | SERVES 4

1 tablespoon real mayonnaise

3 tablespoons nonfat plain yogurt

½ cup nonfat cottage cheese

½ teaspoon cider vinegar

1 teaspoon brown sugar

1 teaspoon Dijon mustard

½ cup buttermilk

2 tablespoons dried parsley

1 clove garlic, minced

2 tablespoons grated Parmesan cheese

¼ teaspoon sea salt (optional)

¼ teaspoon freshly ground pepper (optional)

1 cup chopped cooked chicken breast

½ cup sliced cucumber

½ cup chopped celery

½ cup sliced carrots

4 cups salad greens

½ cup red onion slices

Fresh parsley for garnish (optional)

1. In blender or food processor, combine mayonnaise, yogurt, cottage cheese, vinegar, brown sugar, mustard, buttermilk, parsley, garlic, cheese, salt, and pepper; process until smooth. Pour over the chicken, cucumber, celery, and carrots. Chill at least 2 hours.

2. To serve, arrange 1 cup of salad greens on each of 4 serving plates. Top each salad with an equal amount of chicken salad. Garnish with red onion slices and fresh parsley, if desired.

Get More Mileage from Your Meals

Leftover Chicken Salad makes great sandwiches. Put it between two slices of bread with lots of lettuce for a quick lunch. The lettuce helps keep the bread from getting soggy if the sandwich is to go.

Easy Chicken Paprikash

PER SERVING, using equal amounts of light and dark meat chicken: Calories: 376 | Protein: 22g
Carbohydrates: 58g | Fat: 6g | Saturated Fat: 2g | Cholesterol: 78mg | Sodium: 135mg | Fiber: 4g | PCF Ratio: 23-62-15
Exchange Approx.: ½ Very Lean Meat, ½ Lean Meat, 2½ Starches, 1 Vegetable, 1 Skim Milk

INGREDIENTS | SERVES 4

1 recipe Condensed Cream of Chicken Soup (page 122)

½ cup skim milk

2 teaspoons paprika

⅛ teaspoon ground red pepper (optional)

¼ pound (4 ounces) chopped cooked boneless, skinless chicken

1½ cups sliced steamed mushrooms

½ cup diced steamed onion

½ cup nonfat plain yogurt

4 cups cooked medium-sized egg noodles

1. In saucepan, combine soup, skim milk, paprika, and pepper (if using); whisk until well mixed. Bring to a boil over medium heat, stirring occasionally.

2. Reduce heat to low and stir in chicken, mushrooms, and onion; cook until chicken and vegetables are heated through, about 10 minutes. Stir in yogurt.

3. To serve, put 1 cup of warm, cooked noodles on each of 4 plates. Top each portion with an equal amount of chicken mixture. Garnish by sprinkling with additional paprika, if desired.

For Best Results . . .

Mock condensed soup recipes are used in the dishes in this book so that you know the accurate information. In all cases, you can substitute commercial canned condensed soups; however, be sure to use the lower-fat and lower sodium varieties.

Chicken and Broccoli Casserole

PER SERVING: Calories: 328 | Protein: 26g | Carbohydrates: 20g | Fat: 17g | Saturated Fat: 6g Cholesterol: 67mg | Sodium: 254mg | Fiber: 3g | PCF Ratio: 31-24-45 | Exchange Approx.: 1 Very-Lean Meat, 1 Lean Meat, ½ High-Fat Meat, 1 Fat, 1 Vegetable, 1 Skim Milk, ½ Starch

INGREDIENTS | SERVES 4

2 cups broccoli

½ pound (8 ounces) cooked chopped chicken

½ cup skim milk

⅛ cup (2 tablespoons) real mayonnaise

¼ teaspoon curry powder

1 recipe Condensed Cream of Chicken Soup (page 122)

1 tablespoon lemon juice

½ cup (2 ounces) grated Cheddar cheese

½ cup bread crumbs

1 teaspoon melted butter

1 teaspoon olive oil

1. Preheat oven to 350°F. Treat 11" x 7" casserole dish with nonstick spray.

2. Steam broccoli until tender; drain.

3. Spread out chicken on bottom of dish; cover with steamed broccoli.

4. In medium bowl, combine milk, mayonnaise, curry powder, soup, and lemon juice; pour over broccoli.

5. In small bowl, mix together cheese, bread crumbs, butter, and oil; sprinkle over top of casserole. Bake 30 minutes.

Chicken and Green Bean Stovetop Casserole

PER SERVING: Calories: 305 | Protein: 23g | Carbohydrates: 36g | Fat: 8g | Saturated Fat: 2g | Cholesterol: 48mg
Sodium: 101mg | Fiber: 6g | PCF Ratio: 30-46-24 | Exchange Approx.: 1 Very-Lean Meat, 1 Lean Meat,
1 Vegetable, 1 Starch, 1 Skim Milk

INGREDIENTS | SERVES 4

1 recipe Condensed Cream of Chicken Soup (page 122)

¼ cup skim milk

2 teaspoons Worcestershire sauce (recipe for homemade on page 192)

1 teaspoon real mayonnaise

½ teaspoon onion powder

¼ teaspoon garlic powder

¼ teaspoon ground black pepper

1 (4-ounce) can sliced water chestnuts, drained

2½ cups frozen green beans, thawed

1 cup sliced mushrooms, steamed

½ pound (8 ounces) cooked chopped chicken

1⅓ cups cooked brown long-grain rice

1. Combine soup, milk, Worcestershire, mayonnaise, onion powder, garlic powder, and pepper in a saucepan; bring to a boil.

2. Reduce heat; add water chestnuts, green beans, mushrooms, and chicken. Simmer until vegetables and chicken are heated through, about 10 minutes. Serve over rice.

Veggie Filler

Steamed mushrooms are a low-calorie way to add flavor to a dish and "stretch" the meat. If you don't like mushrooms, you can substitute an equal amount of other low-calorie steamed vegetables like red and green peppers and not significantly affect the total calories in a recipe.

Chicken Pasta with Herb Sauce

PER SERVING: Calories: 393 | Protein: 26g | Carbohydrates: 52g | Fat: 8g | Saturated Fat: 2g | Cholesterol: 48mg
Sodium: 71mg | Fiber: 4g | PCF Ratio: 27-53-20 | Exchange Approx.: 2 Lean Meats, 3 Starches, ½ Skim Milk

INGREDIENTS | SERVES 4

1 recipe Condensed Cream of Chicken Soup (page 122)

¼ cup skim milk

½ teaspoon Worcestershire sauce (recipe for homemade on page 192)

1 teaspoon real mayonnaise

¼ cup grated Parmesan cheese

¼ teaspoon chili powder

½ teaspoon garlic powder

¼ teaspoon dried rosemary

¼ teaspoon dried thyme

¼ teaspoon dried marjoram

1 cup sliced mushrooms, steamed

½ pound (8 ounces) cooked chopped chicken

4 cups cooked pasta

Freshly ground black pepper (optional)

1. Combine soup, milk, Worcestershire, mayonnaise, and cheese in saucepan; bring to a boil.

2. Reduce heat and add chili powder, garlic powder, rosemary, thyme, and marjoram; stir well. Add mushrooms and chicken; simmer for 10 minutes until heated through.

3. Serve over pasta and top with freshly ground pepper, if desired.

Chicken and Asparagus in White Wine Sauce

PER SERVING: Calories: 186 | Protein: 21g | Carbohydrates: 7g | Fat: 8g | Saturated Fat: 2g | Cholesterol: 51mg
Sodium: 57mg | Fiber: 2g | PCF Ratio: 46-16-38 | Exchange Approx.: 2½ Very-Lean Meats, 1½ Vegetables, 1 Fat

INGREDIENTS | SERVES 4

4 boneless, skinless chicken breast halves

½ tablespoon butter

1 tablespoon olive oil

1 teaspoon garlic, finely chopped

½ cup onion, finely chopped

10 ounces asparagus spears, cut diagonally in 2" pieces

½ pound mushrooms

¼ cup dry white wine

¼ cup water

1 tablespoon parsley, chopped

1. Pound chicken pieces to ¼" thickness.

2. Melt butter and olive oil in a large skillet over medium heat. Add chopped garlic and onions; sauté 1–2 minutes.

3. Add chicken; cook 5 minutes, or until the chicken is brown on both sides. Remove chicken and set aside.

4. Add asparagus and mushrooms to skillet; cook 2–3 minutes.

5. Return chicken to skillet; add white wine and water. Bring to a quick boil; boil 2 minutes to reduce the liquid.

6. Reduce heat; cover and simmer 3 minutes, or until chicken and vegetables are tender. Add chopped parsley, salt and pepper to taste, and serve.

Chicken Kalamata

PER SERVING: Calories: 311 | Protein: 31g | Carbohydrates: 25g | Fat: 11g | Saturated Fat: 2g
Cholesterol: 66mg | Sodium: 787mg | Fiber: 6g | PCF Ratio: 38-31-31 | Exchange Approx.: 4 Lean Meats,
2 Vegetables, 1 Starch, 2 Fats

INGREDIENTS | SERVES 4

2 tablespoons olive oil

1 cup onion, chopped

1 teaspoon garlic, minced

1½ cups green peppers, chopped

1 pound boneless, skinless chicken breast, cut into 4 pieces

2 cups tomatoes, diced

1 teaspoon oregano

½ cup pitted kalamata olives, chopped

1. Heat olive oil over medium heat in large skillet. Add onions, garlic, and peppers; sauté for about 5 minutes until onions are translucent.

2. Add chicken pieces; cook for about 5 minutes each side until lightly brown.

3. Add tomatoes and oregano. Reduce heat and simmer 20 minutes.

4. Add olives; simmer an additional 10 minutes before serving.

Are Olives Counted as a Fruit or Vegetable?

The short answer is: neither! Even though olives are a fruit that grows on trees, their flesh is filled with a significant amount of oil and therefore is counted as a fat. Nine black olives or ten green olives equals 1 Fat Serving. The health benefits of olives (and olive oil) comes from the monounsaturated fats they contain. Olives are usually cured in a brine, salt, or olive oil, so if you must watch your salt intake, be careful how many you eat.

Chicken Thighs Cacciatore

PER SERVING: Calories: 370 | Protein: 19g | Carbohydrates: 48g | Fat: 9g | Saturated Fat: 2g | Cholesterol: 39mg
Sodium: 166mg | Fiber: 4g | PCF Ratio: 21-55-24 | Exchange Approx.: 1½ Lean Meats, 2½ Starches,
1 Fat, 1 Vegetable

INGREDIENTS | SERVES 4

2 teaspoons olive oil

½ cup chopped onion

2 cloves garlic, minced

4 chicken thighs, skin removed

½ cup dry red wine

1 (14½-ounce) can unsalted diced tomatoes, undrained

1 teaspoon dried parsley

½ teaspoon dried oregano

¼ teaspoon pepper

⅛ teaspoon sugar

¼ cup grated Parmesan cheese

4 cups cooked spaghetti

2 teaspoons extra-virgin olive oil

1. Heat deep, nonstick skillet over medium-high heat; add 2 teaspoons olive oil. Add onion; sauté until transparent. Add garlic and chicken thighs; sauté 3 minutes on each side, or until lightly browned.

2. Remove thighs from pan; add wine, tomatoes and juices, parsley, oregano, pepper, and sugar. Stir well, bring to a boil. Add chicken back to pan; sprinkle Parmesan cheese over top. Cover, reduce heat, and simmer 10 minutes. Uncover and simmer 10 more minutes.

3. To serve, put 1 cup of cooked pasta on each of 4 plates. Top each serving with a chicken thigh; divide sauce between dishes. Drizzle ½ teaspoon extra-virgin olive oil over top of each dish and serve.

For Cheese Lovers!

Indulge your love of extra cheese and still have a main dish that's under 400 calories. Prepare Chicken Thighs Cacciatore according to recipe instructions. Top each portion with 1 tablespoon freshly grated Parmesan cheese. With cheese, analysis is: Calories: 398.22; Protein: 21.39g; Carbohydrates: 48.43g; Fat: 11.15g; Saturated Fat: 62g; Cholesterol: 487mg; Sodium: 2814mg; Fiber: 81g; PCF Ratio: 23-51-26; Exchange Approx.: 2 Lean Meats, 2½ Starches, 1 Fat, 1 Vegetable.

Chicken with Portobello Mushrooms and Roasted Garlic

PER SERVING: Calories: 335 | Protein: 26g | Carbohydrates: 39g | Fat: 10g | Saturated Fat: 4g | Cholesterol: 56mg
Sodium: 261mg | Fiber: 3g | PCF Ratio: 30-45-25 | Exchange Approx.: 2½ Lean Meats, ½ Fat, 8 Vegetables

INGREDIENTS | SERVES 4

1 tablespoon olive oil

4 boneless, skinless chicken breasts

1 cup reduced-sodium chicken broth

1 bulb garlic, dry roasted (page 26) and mashed into paste

1 tablespoon butter

2 cups portobello mushrooms, chopped

½ teaspoon thyme

2 tablespoons feta cheese, crumbled

1. Heat olive oil in large nonstick skillet; brown chicken breasts on both sides over medium heat, about 5 minutes per side. Add chicken broth and roasted garlic paste to pan; cover and simmer on low 10 minutes.

2. Meanwhile, sauté mushrooms and thyme in butter in separate, smaller saucepan. Simmer 2 minutes.

3. Add the mushrooms and thyme mixture to the chicken and simmer for an additional 2 minutes.

4. When serving, top each chicken breast with 1½ teaspoons feta cheese and pour sauce over the top.

Chipotle Chicken Wrap

PER SERVING: Calories: 284 | Protein: 24g | Carbohydrates: 28g | Fat: 8g | Saturated Fat: 2g | Cholesterol: 40mg
Sodium: 415mg | Fiber: 2g | PCF Ratio: 35-41-25 | Exchange Approx.: 2 Starches, ½ Vegetable, 3 Lean Meats

INGREDIENTS | SERVES 4

12 ounces boneless, skinless chicken breast

1 tablespoon lime juice

1 tablespoon olive oil

1 teaspoon chipotle seasoning

⅛ teaspoon fresh ground pepper

4 whole-wheat tortillas

½ cup jar salsa

1 cup lettuce, chopped

1. Cut chicken into ½" strips. Place chicken, lime juice, olive oil, chipotle seasoning, and pepper in dish; mix well. Cover and allow chicken to marinate 1 hour.

2. Heat outdoor grill. Wrap tortillas in aluminum foil and place on top rack. Cook chicken strips 7–9 minutes until done, turning strips once during cooking.

3. When ready to make wraps, place chicken strips in center of each heated tortilla, add 2 tablespoons salsa to each, top with chopped lettuce, and wrap.

What Is Chipotle?

A chipotle (chee-POTE-lay) is a smoke-dried jalapeño chili used in Mexican or Tex-Mex dishes. You can purchase dried chipotle peppers or a seasoning mix with chipotle peppers added. Mrs. Dash has a Southwest Chipotle Seasoning blend that is salt free!

Stovetop Grilled Turkey Breast

PER SERVING: Calories: 207 | Protein: 31g | Carbohydrates: 2g | Fat: 8g | Saturated Fat: 2g | Cholesterol: 85mg
Sodium: 68mg | Fiber: 0g | PCF Ratio: 62-3-35 | Exchange Approx.: 4 Very-Lean Meats, ½ Fat

INGREDIENTS | SERVES 4

1 teaspoon cider vinegar

1 teaspoon garlic powder

1 teaspoon Dijon mustard

1 teaspoon brown sugar

¼ teaspoon black pepper

2 teaspoons olive oil

4 (4-ounce) turkey breast cutlets

Tip

Cutlets prepared this way tend to cook faster than on an outdoor grill. If using an indoor grill that cooks both sides at once, allow 4–5 minutes total cooking time. You can also use a well seasoned cast-iron skillet instead of a grill pan; however, you may need to introduce more oil to the pan to prevent the cutlets from sticking. Cooking time will be the same as with a grill pan. Be sure to adjust the Fat Exchange, if necessary.

1. In a medium bowl, combine vinegar, garlic powder, mustard, brown sugar, and black pepper; slowly whisk in olive oil to thoroughly combine and make a thin paste.

2. Rinse turkey cutlets and dry thoroughly on paper towels. If necessary to ensure a uniform thickness, put between sheets of plastic wrap and pound to flatten.

3. Pour paste into heavy-duty freezer-style resealable plastic bag. Add cutlets, moving around in mixture to coat all sides. Seal bag, carefully squeezing out as much air as possible. Refrigerate to allow turkey to marinate at least 1 hour, or as long as overnight.

4. Place nonstick hard-anodized stovetop grill pan over high heat. When pan is heated thoroughly, add cutlets. Lower heat to medium-high; cook cutlets 3 minutes on 1 side. Use tongs to turn; cook another 3 minutes, or until juices run clean.

Turkey Mushroom Burgers

PER SERVING: Calories: 100 | Protein: 15g | Carbohydrates: 3g | Fat: 3g | Saturated Fat: 1g | Cholesterol: 34mg
Sodium: 36mg | Fiber: 1g | PCF Ratio: 60-10-30 | Exchange Approx.: 1 Lean Meat, 1 Vegetable, ½ Fat

INGREDIENTS | YIELDS 8 LARGE BURGERS

1 pound turkey breast

1 pound fresh button mushrooms

1 tablespoon olive oil

1 teaspoon butter

1 clove garlic, minced

1 tablespoon green onion, chopped

¼ teaspoon dried thyme

¼ teaspoon dried oregano

¼ teaspoon freshly ground black pepper

Cayenne pepper or dried red pepper flakes, to taste (optional)

1. Cut turkey into even pieces about 1" square. Place cubes in freezer 10 minutes, or long enough to allow turkey to become somewhat firm.

2. In a covered microwave-safe container, microwave mushrooms on high 3–4 minutes, or until they begin to soften and sweat. Set aside to cool slightly.

3. Process turkey in food processor until ground, scraping down sides of bowl as necessary. Add oil, butter, garlic, onion, and mushrooms (and any resulting liquid from the mushrooms); process until mushrooms are ground, scraping down sides of bowl as necessary. Add remaining ingredients; pulse until mixed. Shape into 8 equal-sized patties. Cooking times will vary according to method used and how thick burgers are.

Turkey Marsala with Fresh Peas

PER SERVING: Calories: 278 | Protein: 30g | Carbohydrates: 14g | Fat: 7g | Saturated Fat: 3g
Cholesterol: 78mg | Sodium: 208mg | Fiber: 2g | PCF Ratio: 50-24-27 | Exchange Approx.:
4 Very-Lean Meats, ½ Starch, ½ Vegetable, 1 Fat

INGREDIENTS | SERVES 4

¼ cup all-purpose flour

¼ teaspoon salt

¼ teaspoon pepper

½ teaspoon paprika

1 pound raw turkey breast cutlets, sliced ¼" thick

1 tablespoon olive oil

1 tablespoon butter

½ cup onion, thinly sliced

½ cup Marsala wine

½ cup fresh or frozen peas

1. In a plastic zip-top bag, mix together flour, salt, pepper, and paprika. Place turkey cutlets in plastic bag; shake to coat cutlets with flour.

2. Heat olive and butter in large skillet; sauté onions for about 5 minutes, until browned. Add coated turkey cutlets; brown on both sides, approximately 7–8 minutes on each side.

3. Add Marsala to pan; stir well to combine. Bring to a boil; reduce heat. Turn cutlets to coat both sides.

4. Add peas; continue to cook, stirring, another 2–3 minutes. Serve.

Quick Tip

It's easy to prepare quick and healthy meals if you keep skinless, boneless chicken or turkey in the freezer. If you use an indoor grill, you don't even need to thaw them first. You can prepare a quick sauce or glaze in the time it takes for the chicken or turkey to cook.

Honey and Cider Glaze for Baked Chicken

PER SERVING, glaze only: Calories: 10 | Protein: 0g | Carbohydrates: 2g | Fat: 0g | Saturated Fat: 0g
Cholesterol: 0mg | Sodium: 55mg | Fiber: 0g | PCF Ratio: 9-90-1 | Exchange Approx.: 1 Free Condiment

INGREDIENTS | SERVES 4

3 tablespoons cider or apple juice
½ teaspoon honey
1 teaspoon lemon juice
1 teaspoon Bragg's Liquid Aminos
½ teaspoon lemon zest

Spice Tea Chicken Marinade

Steep 4 orange or lemon spice tea bags in 2 cups boiling water for 4 minutes. Dissolve 1 teaspoon honey into the tea, pour it over 4 chicken pieces, and marinate for 30 minutes. Occasionally turn and baste any exposed portions of chicken. Pour the tea into the roasting pan to provide moisture—discard it after cooking.

1. Preheat oven to 375°F. Combine all ingredients in microwave-safe bowl; microwave on high 30 seconds. Stir until honey is dissolved.

2. To use glaze, arrange 4 boneless chicken pieces with skin removed on rack placed in roasting pan or broiling pan. Brush or spoon 1 teaspoon of glaze over top of each piece. Baste halfway through cooking time, and again 5 minutes before chicken is done. Allow chicken to sit 5 minutes before serving.

CHAPTER 7

Fish and Seafood

Slow-Roasted Salmon

PER SERVING: Calories: 257 | Protein: 25g | Carbohydrates: 1g | Fat: 16g | Saturated Fat: 3g
Cholesterol: 710mg | Sodium: 69mg | Fiber: 1g | PCF Ratio: 41-1-59 | Exchange Approx.: 4 Lean Meats, ½ Fat

INGREDIENTS | SERVES 4

2 teaspoons extra-virgin olive oil

4 (5-ounce) salmon fillets with skin, room temperature

1 cup finely minced fresh chives

Sea or kosher salt and freshly ground white pepper, to taste (optional)

Sage sprigs, for garnish

1. Preheat oven to 250°F. Rub ½ teaspoon of olive oil into flesh side of each salmon fillet. Completely cover fillets with chives; gently press into flesh. Season with salt and pepper, if desired.

2. Place fillets skin-side down on nonstick oven-safe skillet or foil-lined cookie sheet treated with nonstick spray; roast 25 minutes.

Salmon Patties

PER SERVING: Calories: 168 | Protein: 17g | Carbohydrates: 3g | Fat: 9g | Saturated Fat: 2g | Cholesterol: 70mg
Sodium: 92mg | Fiber: 0g | PCF Ratio: 42-8-50 | Exchange Approx.: 2 Lean Meats, ½ Fat, ½ Starch

INGREDIENTS | SERVES 5

2 cups flaked cooked salmon (no salt added)

6 soda crackers, crushed

1 egg

½ cup skim milk

1 small onion, chopped

1 tablespoon fresh parsley, chopped

1 tablespoon unbleached all-purpose flour

1 tablespoon olive oil

Ener-G rice flour (optional)

1. Place salmon in a bowl; flake with fork. Add crushed crackers, egg, milk, onion, parsley, and flour; mix well. Gently form 5 patties.

2. Heat oil in nonstick skillet over medium heat. (Optional: Lightly dust patties with some Ener-G rice flour for crispier patties.) Fry on both sides until browned, about 5 minutes per side.

A-Taste-of-Italy Baked Fish

PER SERVING: Calories: 128 | Protein: 22g | Carbohydrates: 7g | Fat: 1g | Saturated Fat: 0g | Cholesterol: 50mg Sodium: 312mg | Fiber: 1g | PCF Ratio: 68-23-9 | Exchange Approx.: 2½ Very-Lean Meats, 1½ Vegetables

INGREDIENTS | SERVES 4

1 pound (16 ounces) cod fillets
1 (14½-ounce) can stewed tomatoes
¼ teaspoon dried minced onion
½ teaspoon dried minced garlic
¼ teaspoon dried basil
¼ teaspoon dried parsley
⅛ teaspoon dried oregano
⅛ teaspoon sugar
1 tablespoon grated Parmesan cheese

1. Preheat oven to 375°F. Rinse cod with cold water and pat dry with paper towels.

2. In medium-sized baking pan or casserole treated with nonstick cooking spray, combine all ingredients except fish; mix.

3. Arrange fillets over mixture, folding thin tail ends under; spoon mixture over fillets. For fillets about 1" thick, bake uncovered 20–25 minutes, or until fish is opaque and flaky.

Crab Cakes with Sesame Crust

PER SERVING: Calories: 108 | Protein: 9g | Carbohydrates: 3g | Fat: 6g | Saturated Fat: 1g | Cholesterol: 45mg Sodium: 171mg | Fiber: 1g | PCF Ratio: 34-11-55 | Exchange Approx.: 1 Very-Lean Meat, 1½ Fats

INGREDIENTS | SERVES 5

1 pound (16 ounces) lump crabmeat
1 egg
1 tablespoon fresh ginger, minced
1 small scallion, finely chopped
1 tablespoon dry sherry
1 tablespoon freshly squeezed lemon juice
6 tablespoons real mayonnaise
Sea salt and freshly ground white pepper, to taste (optional)
Old Bay Seasoning (Appendix C), to taste (optional)
¼ cup lightly toasted sesame seeds

1. Preheat oven to 375°F. In large bowl, mix together crab, egg, ginger, scallion, sherry, lemon juice, mayonnaise, and seasonings, if using.

2. Form the mixture into 10 equal cakes. Spread sesame seeds over sheet pan; dip both sides of cakes to coat them. Arrange cakes on baking sheet treated with nonstick spray. Typical baking time is 8–10 minutes, depending on thickness of cakes.

Grilled Haddock with Peach-Mango Salsa

PER SERVING, including ½ cup peach-mango salsa: Calories: 204 | Protein: 22g | Carbohydrates: 11g
Fat: 8g | Saturated Fat: 1g | Cholesterol: 65mg | Sodium: 467mg | Fiber: 2g | PCF Ratio: 43-22-35 | Exchange
Approx.: 3 Very-Lean Meats, 1 Fat, ½ Fruit

INGREDIENTS | SERVES 4

1 pound haddock fillets
2 tablespoons olive oil
2 tablespoons lime juice
¼ teaspoon salt
¼ teaspoon ground pepper
1 pound haddock fillets
Peach-Mango Salsa (page 187)

1. Mix olive oil, lime juice, salt, and pepper in a shallow dish; add haddock. Turn and coat fish with marinade.

2. Heat gas grill or broiler. Spray large piece of aluminum foil with nonstick cooking spray. Place fillets on foil; cook 7–8 minutes on each side, or until fish is tender when pierced with a fork.

3. Top each piece of fish with ½ cup fresh Peach-Mango Salsa.

Sesame Shrimp and Asparagus

PER SERVING: Calories: 257 | Protein: 28g | Carbohydrates: 23g | Fat: 6g | Saturated Fat: 1g | Cholesterol: 172mg
Sodium: 173mg | Fiber: 3g | PCF Ratio: 44-35-21 | Exchange Approx.: 3 Very-Lean Meats, ½ Vegetable, 1 Starch

INGREDIENTS | SERVES 4

2 teaspoons canola oil
2 cloves garlic, chopped
1 tablespoon fresh ginger root, grated
1 pound medium shrimp
2 tablespoons dry white wine
½ pound asparagus, cut diagonally into 1" pieces
2 cups whole-grain pasta, cooked
½ teaspoon sesame seeds
¼ cup scallions, thinly sliced
1 teaspoon sesame oil

1. Heat oil in wok or large nonstick skillet. Stir fry garlic, ginger root, and shrimp over high heat until shrimp begins to turn pink, about 2 minutes.

2. Add white wine and asparagus; stir fry an additional 3–5 minutes.

3. Add pasta, sesame seeds, scallions, and sesame oil; toss lightly and serve.

Fish Stock

PER SERVING: Calories: 40 | Protein: 5g | Carbohydrates: 0g | Fat: 2g | Saturated Fat: 1g | Cholesterol: 2mg
Sodium: Variable | Fiber: 0g | PCF Ratio: 55-0-45 | Exchange Approx.: 1 Very-Lean Meat

**INGREDIENTS | YIELDS 4 CUPS;
SERVING SIZE: 1 CUP**

4 cups fish heads, bones, and trimmings
(approx. 1 pound)
2 stalks celery and leaves, chopped
1 onion, chopped
1 carrot, peeled and chopped
1 bay leaf
4 sprigs fresh parsley
Sea salt and pepper, to taste (optional)

1. Use your own fish trimmings (saved in bag in the freezer) or ask the butcher at your local fish market or supermarket for fish trimmings. Wash the trimmings well.

2. In a stockpot, combine all ingredients; add enough water to cover everything by an inch or so. Bring to a boil over high heat; reduce heat to low. Skim off foam that rises to top. Cover and simmer 20 minutes.

3. Remove from heat; strain through a sieve, discarding all solids. Refrigerate or freeze.

Spicy "Fried" Fish Fillet

PER SERVING: Calories: 230 | Protein: 24g | Carbohydrates: 9g | Fat: 10g | Saturated Fat: 2g | Cholesterol: 116mg
Sodium: 412mg | Fiber: 1g | PCF Ratio: 44-17-39 | Exchange Approx.: 3 Very-Lean Meats, 2 Fats, ½ Starch

INGREDIENTS | SERVES 4

16 ounces flounder, cut into 4 pieces
⅓ cup cornmeal
½ teaspoon salt
1 teaspoon chipotle seasoning
1 egg
2 tablespoons 1% milk
16 ounces flounder, cut into 4 pieces
2 tablespoons olive oil

1. Combine cornmeal, salt, and chipotle seasoning in shallow dish.

2. Beat egg and milk together in shallow dish.

3. Dip fish in egg mixture; coat each fillet with cornmeal mixture.

4. Heat olive oil in nonstick skillet; brown fillets until golden and crispy, about 6–7 minutes each side.

Baked Bread Crumb–Crusted Fish with Lemon

PER SERVING, without salt: Calories: 137 | Protein: 24g | Carbohydrates: 5g | Fat: 3g | Saturated Fat: 1g
Cholesterol: 36mg | Sodium: 73mg | Fiber: 2g | PCF Ratio: 68-14-18 | Exchange Approx.: 2 Very-Lean Meats, ½ Starch, ½ Free Condiment

INGREDIENTS | SERVES 6

2 large lemons

¼ cup dried bread crumbs

1½ pounds (24 ounces) halibut fillets

Sea or kosher salt and freshly ground white or black pepper, to taste (optional)

Lemon Infusion

Mildly flavored fish such as catfish, cod, halibut, orange roughy, rockfish, and snapper benefit from the distinctive flavor of lemon. Adding slices of lemon to top of fish allows the flavor to infuse into fish.

1. Preheat oven to 375°F. Wash 1 lemon; cut into thin slices. Grate 1 tablespoon of zest from the second lemon, then juice it. Combine grated zest and bread crumbs in small bowl; stir to mix. Set aside.

2. Put lemon juice in shallow dish; arrange lemon slices in bottom of baking dish treated with nonstick spray. Dip fish pieces in lemon juice; set on lemon slices in baking dish.

3. Sprinkle bread crumb mixture evenly over fish pieces along with salt and pepper, if using; bake until crumbs are lightly browned and fish is just opaque, 10–15 minutes. (Baking time will depend on thickness of fish.) Serve immediately, using lemon slices as garnish.

Baked Red Snapper Almandine

PER SERVING, without salt: Calories: 178 | Protein: 24g | Carbohydrates: 3g | Fat: 7g | Saturated Fat: 2g
Cholesterol: 47mg | Sodium: 73mg | Fiber: 1g | PCF Ratio: 56-7-37 | Exchange Approx.: 3 Lean Meats

INGREDIENTS | SERVES 4

1 pound (16 ounces) red snapper fillets

Sea or kosher salt and freshly ground white or black pepper, to taste (optional)

4 teaspoons all-purpose flour

2 teaspoons olive oil

2 tablespoons ground raw almonds

2 teaspoons unsalted butter

1 tablespoon lemon juice

1. Preheat oven to 375°F. Rinse red snapper fillets and dry between layers of paper towels. Season with salt and pepper, if using; sprinkle with flour, front and back.

2. In an ovenproof nonstick skillet, sauté fillets in olive oil until nicely browned on both sides, about 5 minutes per side.

3. Combine ground almonds and butter in microwave-safe dish. Microwave on high 30 seconds, or until butter is melted; stir to combine. Pour almond-butter mixture and lemon juice over fillets; bake 3–5 minutes, or until almonds are nicely browned.

Asian-Style Fish Cakes

PER SERVING: Calories: 66 | Protein: 11g | Carbohydrates: 1g | Fat: 2g | Saturated Fat: 1g | Cholesterol: 41mg
Sodium: 112mg | Fiber: 0mg | PCF Ratio: 69-8-23 | Exchange Approx.: 1 Lean Meat, 1 Free Condiment

INGREDIENTS | SERVES 8

1-pound catfish fillet

2 green onions, minced

1 banana pepper, cored, seeded, and chopped

2 cloves garlic, minced

1 tablespoon ginger, grated or minced

1 tablespoon Bragg's Liquid Aminos

1 tablespoon lemon juice

1 teaspoon lemon zest

Old Bay seasoning (Appendix C), optional

Tip

For crunchy fish cakes, coat each side in rice flour and then lightly spritz the tops of the patties with olive or peanut oil before baking as directed.

1. Preheat oven to 375°F. Cut fish into 1" pieces. Combine with green onions, banana pepper, garlic, ginger, Bragg's Liquid Aminos, lemon juice, and lemon zest in food processor; process until chopped and mixed. (You do not want to purée this mixture; it should be a rough chop.) Add Old Bay Seasoning, if using; stir to mix.

2. Form fish mixture into patties of about 2 tablespoons each; you should have 16 patties total. Place patties on baking sheet treated with nonstick cooking spray; bake 12–15 minutes, or until crisp. (Alternatively, you can fry these in a nonstick pan about 4 minutes on each side.)

Creamy Shrimp Pie with Rice Crust

PER SERVING: Calories: 273 | Protein: 26g | Carbohydrates: 27g | Fat: 6g | Saturated Fat: 2g | Cholesterol: 180mg
Sodium: 172mg | Fiber: 2g | PCF Ratio: 39-40-21 | Exchange Approx.: 2 Very-Lean Meats, 2 Starches, 1 Fat

INGREDIENTS | SERVES 4

1⅓ cups cooked white rice

2 teaspoons dried parsley

2 tablespoons grated onion

1 teaspoon olive oil

1 tablespoon butter

1 clove garlic, crushed

1 pound shrimp, peeled and deveined

1 recipe Condensed Cream of Mushroom Soup (page 127)

1 teaspoon lemon juice

1 cup sliced mushrooms, steamed

Fat-Free Flavor

To add the flavor of sautéed mushrooms or onions without the added fat of butter or oil, roast or grill them first. Simply spread them on a baking sheet treated with non-stick spray. Roasting for 5 minutes in a 350°F oven will be sufficient if the vegetables are sliced, and will not add additional cooking time to the recipe.

1. Preheat oven to 350°F. Combine rice, parsley, and onion; mix well. Use olive oil to coat 10" pie plate; press rice mixture evenly around sides and bottom. This works best if the rice is moist; if necessary, add 1 teaspoon of water.

2. Melt butter in deep, nonstick skillet over medium heat; sauté garlic. Add shrimp; cook, stirring frequently, until pink, about 5 minutes.

3. Add soup and lemon juice to skillet; stir until smooth and thoroughly heated, about 5 minutes. (If the soup seems too thick, add some water, 1 teaspoon at a time.) Stir mushrooms into soup mixture; pour over rice "crust." Bake 30 minutes, or until lightly browned on top. Serve hot.

Barley-Spinach-Fish Bake

**PER SERVING: Calories: 239 | Protein: 26g | Carbohydrates: 15g | Fat: 8g | Saturated Fat: 1g
Cholesterol: 67mg | Sodium: 418mg | Fiber: 3g | PCF Ratio: 44-26-30 | Exchange Approx.:
3 Lean Meats, ½ Starch, 1 Vegetable, 1½ Fats**

INGREDIENTS | SERVES 4

½ tablespoon olive oil

¼ cup scallions, chopped

1 clove garlic, minced

¼ teaspoon rosemary

¼ teaspoon marjoram

¼ teaspoon salt

1 cup pearl barley, cooked

5 ounces (½ box) frozen chopped spinach, thawed and drained

¼ cup sundried tomatoes, chopped

4 (12-inch) squares of aluminum foil

4 (4-ounce) fish fillets

3 tablespoons white wine

Salt and fresh ground pepper, to taste

1. Preheat oven to 400°F (or outdoor grill can be used).

2. Heat oil in medium nonstick skillet; add scallions and sauté 2 minutes. Add garlic, rosemary, marjoram, and salt; continue to cook another 3 minutes, until scallions are tender. Add cooked barley, spinach, and sundried tomatoes; mix well.

3. Place aluminum foil squares on work surface; place a fish fillet in center of each square. Divide barley mixture equally; place on top of each fillet. Sprinkle with white wine, salt, and pepper.

4. Fold aluminum foil loosely to enclose filling. Place packets on baking sheet (or directly on grill if using outdoor grill); bake 15 minutes, or until fish is tender and flakes easily.

Cooking Barley

Pearl barley takes longer to cook than quick-cooking barley, so you will want to prepare it in advance. To prepare: Bring ½ cup pearl barley and 1 cup water to a boil. Reduce heat, cover, and simmer for 35–45 minutes, or until all water is absorbed. Pearl barley makes a good side dish on its own with the addition of spices or vegetables.

Grilled Salmon with Roasted Peppers

PER SERVING: Calories: 269 | Protein: 24g | Carbohydrates: 8g | Fat: 16g | Saturated Fat: 3g | Cholesterol: 67mg
Sodium: 321mg | Fiber: 1g | PCF Ratio: 36-11-53 | Exchange Approx.: 3½ Lean Meats, 1 Vegetable, 1 Fat

INGREDIENTS | SERVES 4

4 (4-ounce) salmon steaks
1 tablespoon reduced-sodium soy sauce
1 tablespoon brown sugar
1 tablespoon olive oil
2 large red bell peppers
1 tablespoon balsamic vinegar
½ teaspoon dried thyme
¼ teaspoon fresh-ground pepper

Wasabi Marinade

Wasabi, also known as Japanese horserad-ish, can be purchased in raw form or as a powder or paste. It adds a hot, pungent flavor to fish and works especially well with salmon. To make a marinade for salmon or other fish, mix 1 teaspoon wasabi powder (or paste) with 2 tablespoons low-sodium soy sauce, ½ teaspoon grated ginger, and 1 teaspoon sesame oil. Coat fish with the marinade and grill.

1. Place salmon in shallow dish. Mix together soy sauce, brown sugar, and olive oil; pour over salmon and cover both sides with marinade. Set aside.

2. Prepare roasted red peppers following procedure on page 196. Once peppers are roasted and peeled, cut into strips and sprinkle balsamic vinegar, thyme, and pepper. Set aside.

3. Heat grill. Remove salmon from the marinade; grill over medium heat approximately 8 minutes on one side. Turn and grill on other side until salmon is cooked and tender, about 4–5 minutes longer. Remove from heat.

4. Top each salmon steak with marinated roasted red peppers.

Baked Snapper with Orange-Rice Dressing

PER SERVING, without salt: Calories: 257 | Protein: 26g | Carbohydrates: 25g | Fat: 5g | Saturated Fat: 2g
Cholesterol: 47mg | Sodium: 83mg | Fiber: 1g | PCF Ratio: 41-40-19 | Exchange Approx.: 2 Lean Meats,
½ Fruit, ½ Fat, 1 Starch

INGREDIENTS | SERVES 4

¼ cup chopped celery

½ cup chopped onion

½ cup orange juice

1 tablespoon lemon juice

1 teaspoon grated orange zest

1⅓ cups cooked rice

1 pound (16 ounces) red snapper fillets

Sea or kosher salt and freshly ground white or black pepper, to taste (optional)

2 teaspoons unsalted butter

2 tablespoons ground raw almonds

1. Preheat oven to 350°F.

2. In a microwave-safe bowl, mix celery and onion with juices and orange zest; microwave on high 2 minutes, or until mixture comes to a boil. Add rice; stir to moisten, adding water 1 tablespoon at a time if necessary to thoroughly coat rice. Cover and let stand 5 minutes.

3. Rinse fillets and pat dry between paper towels. Prepare baking dish with nonstick spray. Spread rice mixture in dish; arrange fillets on top. Season fillets with salt and pepper, if using.

4. Combine butter and almonds in a microwave-safe bowl; microwave on high 30 seconds, or until butter is melted. Stir; spoon over top of fillets.

5. Cover and bake 10 minutes. Remove cover and bake another 5–10 minutes, or until fish flakes easily when tested with a fork and almonds are lightly browned.

Crunchy "Fried" Catfish Fillets

**PER SERVING, without salt: Calories: 244 | Protein: 21g | Carbohydrates: 18g | Fat: 9g | Saturated Fat: 2g
Cholesterol: 53mg | Sodium: 248mg | Fiber: 1g | PCF Ratio: 35-30-35 | Exchange Approx.: 3 Lean Meats, 1 Starch**

INGREDIENTS | SERVES 4

1 egg white (from a large egg), room temperature

¼ cup bread crumbs

¼ cup enriched white cornmeal

1 teaspoon grated lemon zest

½ teaspoon crushed dried basil

¼ cup all-purpose flour

⅛ teaspoon kosher or sea salt (optional)

¼ teaspoon lemon pepper

Zesty Crunch

Grated lemon or lime zest is a great way to give added citrus flavor to a crunchy bread-crumb topping for fish.

1. Preheat oven to 450°F; treat shallow baking pan with nonstick spray. Rinse catfish and dry between layers of paper towels.

2. In shallow dish, beat egg white until frothy. In another dish, combine bread crumbs, cornmeal, lemon zest, and basil. In third dish, combine flour, salt (if using), and lemon pepper.

3. Dip fish into flour mixture to coat 1 side of each fillet. Shake off any excess flour mixture, then dip flour-covered side of fillet into egg white. Next, coat covered side of fillet with bread-crumb mixture.

4. Arrange prepared fillets side by side, coated-sides up, on prepared baking pan. Tuck in any thin edges. Bake 6–12 minutes, or until fish flakes easily with a fork.

Baked Orange Roughy with Spicy Plum Sauce

PER SERVING: Calories: 221 | Protein: 19g | Carbohydrates: 31g | Fat: 3g | Saturated Fat: 1g | Cholesterol: 23mg
Sodium: 101mg | Fiber: 2g | PCF Ratio: 34-56-11 | Exchange Approx.: 2 Very-Lean Meats, 1 Fruit, 1 Starch

INGREDIENTS | SERVES 4

1 pound (16 ounces) orange roughy fillets

1 teaspoon paprika

1 bay leaf

1 clove garlic, crushed

1 apple, peeled, cored, and cubed

1 teaspoon grated fresh ginger

1 small red or Spanish onion, chopped

1 teaspoon olive oil

¼ cup Plum Sauce (page 196)

¼ teaspoon Chinese five spice powder

1 teaspoon frozen unsweetened apple juice concentrate

½ teaspoon Bragg's Liquid Aminos

¼ teaspoon blackstrap molasses

1⅓ cups cooked brown rice

1. Preheat oven to 400°F. Treat baking dish with nonstick spray. Rinse orange roughy and pat dry between paper towels. Rub both sides of fish with paprika; set in prepared dish.

2. In covered microwave-safe bowl, mix bay leaf, garlic, apple, ginger, and onion in oil; microwave on high 3 minutes, or until apple is tender and onion is transparent. Stir; discard bay leaf and top fillets with mixture. Bake uncovered 15–18 minutes, or until fish is opaque.

3. While fish bakes, add plum sauce to microwave-safe bowl. Add five spice, apple juice concentrate, Liquid Aminos, and molasses. Microwave on high 30 seconds; stir, add a little water if needed to thin mixture, and microwave another 15 seconds. Cover until ready to serve. If necessary, bring back to temperature by microwaving mixture another 15 seconds just prior to serving.

4. To serve, equally divide cooked rice among 4 serving plates. Top each with an equal amount of baked fish and plum sauce, drizzling sauce atop fish.

Jon's Fish Tacos

PER SERVING: Calories: 383 | Protein: 29g | Carbohydrates: 40g | Fat: 12g | Saturated Fat: 2g
Cholesterol: 60mg | Sodium: 400mg | Fiber: 4g | PCF Ratio: 30-42-28 | Exchange Approx.:
3½ Very-Lean Meats, 2 Starches, 1 Vegetable, 1 Fat

INGREDIENTS | SERVES 4

¼ cup light mayonnaise
½ cup plain nonfat yogurt
¼ cup onion, chopped
2 tablespoons jalapeño pepper, minced
2 teaspoons cilantro, minced
2 cups cabbage, shredded
¼ cup lime juice
1 clove garlic, minced
1 tablespoon canola oil
1 pound tilapia fillets
4 whole-wheat tortillas, 6" diameter
Aluminum foil
Nonstick cooking spray
1 cup tomato, chopped

1. In medium bowl, whisk together mayonnaise, yogurt, onion, jalapeño, and cilantro. Stir in shredded cabbage; chill.

2. In separate bowl, combine lime juice, garlic, and canola oil to make a marinade for fish. Pour over fish; cover and refrigerate at least 1 hour.

3. Place fish on aluminum-lined grill (spray aluminum with cooking spray); cook 6–7 minutes on each side, until fish is tender and beginning to flake.

4. While fish is cooking, loosely wrap whole-wheat tortilla in large piece of aluminum foil to heat.

5. To assemble tacos, cut fish into strips; divide into 4 portions. Place strips in center of each heated tortilla. Top with coleslaw mixture and chopped tomatoes. Add fresh ground pepper, if desired.

Sweet Onion–Baked Yellowtail Snapper

PER SERVING, no salt: Calories: 189 | **Protein:** 25g | **Carbohydrates:** 13g | **Fat:** 4g | **Saturated Fat:** 1g
Cholesterol: 42mg | **Sodium:** 77mg | **Fiber:** 1g | **PCF Ratio:** 53-28-19 | **Exchange Approx.:** 1 Lean Meat,
2 Very-Lean Meats, 1 Vegetable, ½ Starch

INGREDIENTS | SERVES 4

2 cups sliced Vidalia onions

1 tablespoon balsamic vinegar

2 teaspoons brown sugar

4 teaspoons olive oil

1 pound (16 ounces) skinless yellowtail snapper fillets

Sea salt and freshly ground white or black pepper, to taste (optional)

1. In covered microwave-safe dish, microwave onion on high 5 minutes, or until transparent. Carefully remove cover; stir in vinegar and brown sugar. Cover; allow to sit several minutes so onion absorbs flavors.

2. Heat a nonstick pan on medium-high; add olive oil. Transfer steamed onion mixture to pan; sauté until browned but not crisp. (Be careful, as onions will burn easily because of brown sugar; if onion browns too quickly, lower heat and add a few tablespoons of water.) Cook until all liquid has evaporated from pan, stirring often. Onions should have a shiny and dark caramelized color. (This can be prepared 2–3 days in advance; store tightly covered in refrigerator.)

3. Preheat oven to 375°F. Rinse snapper in cold water and dry between paper towels. Arrange on baking sheet treated with nonstick spray. Spoon caramelized onions over tops of fillets, pressing to form a light crust over top of fish. Bake 12–15 minutes, or until fish flakes easily with a fork. Serve immediately with Madeira sauce divided on 4 plates with fish placed on top.

Stir-Fried Ginger Scallops with Vegetables

PER SERVING: Calories: 145 | Protein: 22g | Carbohydrates: 8g | Fat: 3g | Saturated Fat: 1g | Cholesterol: 37mg
Sodium: 373mg | Fiber: 2g | PCF Ratio: 61-23-16 | Exchange Approx.: 3 Very-Lean Meats, ½ Vegetable

INGREDIENTS | SERVES 4

1 pound (16 ounces) scallops
1 teaspoon peanut or sesame oil
1 tablespoon chopped fresh ginger
2 cloves garlic, minced
4 scallions, thinly sliced (optional)
1 teaspoon rice wine vinegar
2 teaspoons Bragg's Liquid Aminos
½ cup low-fat reduced-sodium chicken broth
2 cups broccoli florets
1 teaspoon cornstarch
¼ teaspoon toasted sesame oil

1. Rinse scallops and pat dry between layers of paper towels. If necessary, slice scallops so they're uniform size. Set aside.

2. Add peanut oil to heated nonstick deep skillet or wok; sauté ginger, garlic, and scallions if using, 1–2 minutes, being careful ginger doesn't burn. Add vinegar, Liquid Aminos, and broth; bring to a boil. Remove from heat.

3. Place broccoli in large, covered microwave-safe dish; pour chicken broth mixture over top. Microwave on high 3–5 minutes, depending on preference. (Keep in mind that vegetables will continue to steam for a minute or so if cover remains on dish.)

4. Heat skillet or wok over medium-high temperature. Add scallops; sauté 1 minute on each side. (Do scallops in batches if necessary; be careful not to overcook.) Remove scallops from pan when done; set aside. Drain (but do not discard) liquid from broccoli; return liquid to bowl and transfer broccoli to heated skillet or wok. Stir-fry vegetables to bring up to serving temperature.

5. Meanwhile, in small cup or bowl, add enough water to cornstarch to make a slurry or roux. Whisk slurry into reserved broccoli liquid; microwave on high 1 minute. Add toasted sesame oil; whisk again. Pour thickened broth mixture over broccoli; toss to mix. Add scallops back to broccoli mixture; stir-fry over medium heat to return scallops to serving temperature. Serve over rice or pasta; adjust Exchange Approximations accordingly.

Scallops and Shrimp with White Bean Sauce

PER SERVING: Calories: 231 | Protein: 27g | Carbohydrates: 18g | Fat: 4g | Saturated Fat: 1g
Cholesterol: 105mg | Sodium: 217mg | Fiber: 7g | PCF Ratio: 49-34-17 | Exchange Approx.:
3 Very-Lean Meats, ½ Fat, 1 Starch, ½ Vegetable

INGREDIENTS | SERVES 4

½ cup finely chopped onion, steamed

2 cloves garlic, minced

2 teaspoons olive oil, divided

¼ cup dry white wine

¼ cup tightly packed fresh parsley leaves

¼ cup tightly packed fresh basil leaves

1⅓ cups canned cannellini (white) beans, drained and rinsed

¼ cup low-fat, reduced-sodium chicken broth

½ pound (8 ounces) shrimp, shelled and deveined

½ pound (8 ounces) scallops

1. In nonstick saucepan, sauté onion and garlic in 1 teaspoon of oil over moderately low heat, for about 5 minutes until onion is soft. Add wine; simmer until wine is reduced by ½. Add parsley, basil, ⅓ cup of beans, and chicken broth; simmer, stirring constantly for 1 minute.

2. Transfer bean mixture to blender or food processor; purée. Pour purée back into saucepan; add remaining beans; simmer 2 minutes.

3. In nonstick skillet, heat remaining 1 teaspoon of oil over moderately high heat until it is hot but not smoking. Sauté shrimp 2 minutes on each side, or until cooked through. Using slotted spoon, transfer shrimp to plate; cover to keep warm. Add scallops to skillet; sauté 1 minute on each side, or until cooked through. To serve, divide bean sauce between 4 shallow bowls and arrange shellfish over top.

Smoked Mussels and Pasta

PER SERVING: Calories: 206 | Protein: 10g | Carbohydrates: 22g | Fat: 8g | Saturated Fat: 2g
Cholesterol: 31mg | Sodium: 371mg | Fiber: 1g | PCF Ratio: 20-44-35 | Exchange Approx.:
1 Carbohydrate/Starch, 1 Lean Meat, ½ Fat, ½ Skim Milk

INGREDIENTS | SERVES 4

1⅓ cups uncooked pasta (to yield 2 cups cooked pasta)

½ cup chopped leek

4 ounces smoked mussels, drained of all excess oil

⅛ teaspoon cayenne pepper

½ teaspoon dried oregano

¼ cup nonfat cottage cheese

⅛ cup nonfat plain yogurt

2 teaspoons grated Parmesan cheese

2 teaspoons extra-virgin olive oil

Cracked black pepper, to taste

1. Cook pasta according to package directions; drain and set aside. In covered microwave-safe bowl, microwave leek on high 2–3 minutes, or until limp and translucent. Add mussels and cayenne pepper; stir. Cover and microwave on high 30 seconds to heat mussels.

2. In blender, combine oregano, cottage cheese, yogurt, and Parmesan cheese; process until smooth. Combine cottage cheese and mussel mixtures; microwave on high until warm, about 30 seconds. Toss pasta with olive oil; stir in mussel mixture. Divide into 4 portions and serve immediately, topped with cracked pepper.

Savory Smoke

Smoked meats impart a strong, pleasant flavor to dishes, so you can use less meat to achieve a rich taste.

Pasta and Smoked Trout with Lemon Pesto

PER SERVING: Calories: 209 | Protein: 10g | Carbohydrates: 23g | Fat: 8g | Saturated Fat: 1g
Cholesterol: 4mg | Sodium: 151mg | Fiber: 1g | PCF Ratio: 20-45-36 | Exchange Approx.: 1 Fat, 1½
Lean Meats, 1 Carbohydrate/Starch

INGREDIENTS | SERVES 4

2 cloves garlic

2 cups fresh basil leaves, tightly packed

⅛ cup pine nuts, toasted

2 teaspoons fresh lemon juice

2 teaspoons water

4 teaspoons extra-virgin olive oil

4 tablespoons grated Parmesan cheese, divided

1⅓ cups uncooked linguini or other pasta (to yield 2 cups cooked pasta)

2 ounces whole boneless smoked trout

Freshly ground black pepper, to taste

1. Put garlic in food processor; pulse until finely chopped. Add basil, pine nuts, lemon juice, and water; process until just puréed. (Note: You can substitute fresh parsley for basil; supplement flavor by adding some dried basil, too, if you do.) Add olive oil and 3 tablespoons of Parmesan cheese; pulse until pesto is smooth, occasionally scraping down side of bowl, if necessary. Set aside.

2. Cook pasta according to package directions. While it is cooking, flake trout. When pasta is cooked, pulse pesto to ensure it has remained blended; toss pesto and trout with pasta. Sprinkle remaining Parmesan and some pepper on top of each serving. (Although this recipe uses heart-healthy extra-virgin olive oil, it is a little higher in fat, but still low in calories. Consult your dietitian if you have any question whether you should include this recipe in your meal plans.)

Fresh Tomato and Clam Sauce with Whole-Grain Linguini

PER SERVING: Calories: 361 | Protein: 13g | Carbohydrates: 60g | Fat: 8g | Saturated Fat: 1g
Cholesterol: 7mg | Sodium: 356mg | Fiber: 8g | PCF Ratio: 14-66-20 | Exchange Approx.:
2½ Starches, 1½ Very-Lean Meats, 3 Vegetables, 1½ Fats

INGREDIENTS | SERVES 4

3 dozen (36) littleneck clams

2 tablespoons olive oil

5 cloves garlic, chopped

½ cup red bell pepper, chopped

4 cups fresh tomatoes, peeled and chopped

3 tablespoons fresh parsley, chopped

1 tablespoon fresh basil, chopped

¼ teaspoon salt

¼ teaspoon red pepper flakes

½ teaspoon oregano

½ cup dry white wine

8 ounces whole-grain linguini

Tip

This recipe works well with canned clams if you are unable to get fresh. Canned clams are quite high in sodium, which will need to be taken into consideration. If using canned clams, you will need 1 (8-ounce) can of minced clams and 1 (10-ounce) can of whole clams. Reserve the clam juice and add to the sauce.

1. Before preparing this dish (preferably several hours or more), place clams in bowl of cold water with handful of cornmeal added; keep refrigerated. (This will help purge clams of any sand or other debris.) When ready to cook, rinse and scrub clams.

2. Heat olive oil, garlic, and red pepper in a deep skillet. Add chopped tomatoes, parsley, basil, salt, red pepper flakes, and oregano, bring to quick boil, then reduce heat and simmer 15–20 minutes.

3. Stir in white wine; add clams on top of tomato sauce. Cover and steam until clams open. (Discard any clams that do not open; they are not suitable for eating.)

4. Meanwhile, boil water and cook pasta to al dente.

5. Serve tomato sauce and clams over pasta.

Smoked Shrimp and Cheese Quesadillas

PER SERVING: Calories: 272 | Protein: 11g | Carbohydrates: 32g | Fat: 11g | Saturated Fat: 3g
Cholesterol: 39mg | Sodium: 428mg | Fiber: 3g | PCF Ratio: 17-46-37 | Exchange Approx.:
1 Carbohydrate/Starch, 1½ Lean Meats, 1 Fat, ½ Vegetable

INGREDIENTS | SERVES 4

4 (8") flour tortillas

4 teaspoons olive oil

2 ounces part-skim mozzarella or other mild cheese (such as fontina or baby Swiss)

1 jalapeño or banana pepper, finely chopped

2 cloves garlic, crushed

4 ounces smoked shrimp

1 cup thinly sliced red onion

½ cup roughly chopped fresh cilantro

Cut Added Sodium

Reduce sodium content (salty flavor) from smoked seafood like mussels or shrimp by rinsing them in a little water.

1. Preheat oven to 375°F. Lightly brush 1 side of each tortilla with some olive oil. Mix cheese, pepper, and garlic with remaining olive oil; spread ¼ of cheese mixture in center of oiled half of each tortilla. Top with shrimp, red onion, and cilantro; fold tortilla in half to cover ingredients.

2. Place tortillas in baking pan treated with nonstick spray. Bake 3–5 minutes, or until nicely browned and cheese is melted. Serve with your choice of tomato salsa.

CHAPTER 8

Casseroles and Stews

Condensed Cream of Chicken Soup, Minor's Base Method

PER RECIPE: Calories: 158 | Protein: 4g | Carbohydrates: 35g | Fat: 1g | Saturated Fat: 0g
Cholesterol: 1mg | Sodium: 162mg | Fiber: 2g | PCF Ratio: 9-88-3 | Exchange Approx.:
Will depend on serving size and preparation method

INGREDIENTS | YIELDS EQUIVALENT OF 1 (10.75-OUNCE) CAN

1 cup water

¾ teaspoon Minor's Low-Sodium Chicken Base

¼ cup Ener-G potato flour

Place all ingredients in blender; process until well blended.

Condensed Cream of Chicken Soup with Regular Chicken Broth

For the equivalent of 1 (10.75-ounce) can of condensed chicken soup, blend 1 cup reduced-fat canned chicken broth with ¼ cup Ener-G potato flour. Will last, refrigerated, 3 days. Nutritional Analysis: Calories: 181.20; Protein: 61g; Carbohydrates: 314g; Fat: 1.50g; Saturated Fat: 0.42g; Cholesterol: 0.00mg; Sodium: 7820mg; Fiber: 36g; PCF Ratio: 17-76-7; Exchange Approx.: will depend on serving size and preparation method.

Condensed Cream of Celery Soup

PER RECIPE: Calories: 85 | Protein: 2g | Carbohydrates: 20g | Fat: 0g | Saturated Fat: 0g | Cholesterol: 0mg
Sodium: 79mg | Fiber: 2g | PCF Ratio: 9-89-2 | Exchange Approx.: Will depend on
serving size and preparation method

INGREDIENTS | YIELDS EQUIVALENT OF 1 (10.75-OUNCE) CAN

½ cup steamed chopped celery

½ cup water

⅛ cup Ener-G potato flour

1. In a microwave-safe covered container, microwave celery 2 minutes, or until tender. Do not drain any resulting liquid. If necessary, add enough water to bring celery and liquid to 1 cup total.

2. Place all ingredients in blender; process. Use immediately, or store in a covered container in refrigerator for use within 3 days. Thickness of concentrate will depend on how much moisture remains in celery; add 1–2 tablespoons of water, if necessary, to achieve a paste.

Condensed Cream of Potato Soup

PER RECIPE: Calories: 103 | Protein: 2g | Carbohydrates: 24g | Fat: 0g | Saturated Fat: 0g
Cholesterol: 0mg | Sodium: 9mg | Fiber: 2g | PCF Ratio: 8-91-1 | Exchange Approx.:
Will depend on serving size and preparation method

INGREDIENTS | YIELDS EQUIVALENT OF 1 (10.75-OUNCE) CAN

½ cup peeled, diced potatoes

½ cup water

1 tablespoon Ener-G potato flour

Tip

The nutrition information for this recipe assumes you'll use the entire tablespoon of Ener-G potato flour; however, the amount needed will depend on the amount of starch in the potatoes you use. For example, new potatoes will require more Ener-G potato flour than larger, Idaho-style potatoes.

1. Place potatoes and water in covered microwave-safe bowl; microwave on high 4–5 minutes, until potatoes are fork-tender.

2. Pour potatoes and water in blender, being careful of steam. Remove vent from blender lid; process until smooth. Add Ener-G 1 teaspoon at a time while blender is running.

Condensed Cheese Soup

PER RECIPE: Calories: 315 | Protein: 20g | Carbohydrates: 18g | Fat: 18g | Saturated Fat: 11g
Cholesterol: 56mg | Sodium: 384mg | Fiber: 1g | PCF Ratio: 26-23-51 | Exchange Approx.:
Will depend on serving size and preparation method

INGREDIENTS | YIELDS EQUIVALENT OF 1 (10.75-OUNCE) CAN

½ cup water

⅛ cup Ener-G potato flour

¼ cup nonfat cottage cheese

2 ounces American, Cheddar, or Colby cheese, shredded (to yield ½ cup)

Place water, potato flour, and cottage cheese in blender; process until well blended. Stir in shredded cheese. Cheese will melt as casserole is baked, prepared in microwave, or cooked on stovetop, according to recipe instructions.

Be Aware of Your Exchanges

When using any soup preparation method, you'll need to add the appropriate Exchange Approximations for each serving amount (usually ¼ of the total) of whatever condensed soup you make. For example, broth-based soups like chicken and cream of mushroom or celery would be a Free Exchange; cream of potato soup would add 1 Carbohydrate/Starch.

Condensed Tomato Soup

PER SERVING: Calories: 136 | Protein: 4g | Carbohydrates: 31g | Fat: 1g | Saturated Fat: 0g
Cholesterol: 0mg | Sodium: 352mg | Fiber: 4g | PCF Ratio: 11-83-6 | Exchange Approx.:
Will depend on serving size and preparation method

INGREDIENTS | YIELDS EQUIVALENT OF 1 (10.75-OUNCE) CAN

1 cup peeled chopped tomato, with juice
Additional tomato juices (if necessary)
¼ teaspoon baking soda
⅛ cup Ener-G potato flour

1. Place tomato in microwave-safe bowl; microwave on high 2–3 minutes, until tomato is cooked. Add additional tomato juices if necessary to bring mixture back up to 1 cup.

2. Add baking soda; stir vigorously until bubbling stops.

3. Pour cooked tomato mixture into blender; add potato flour, 1 tablespoon at a time, processing until well blended.

Direct Preparation

If you'll be making the soup immediately after you prepare the condensed soup recipe, you can simply add your choice of the additional 1 cup of liquid (such as skim milk, soy milk, or water) to the blender and use that method to mix the milk and soup concentrate together. Pour the combined mixture into your pan or microwave-safe dish.

Soup Preparation Method

PER SERVING, skim milk: Additional Calories: 21 | Protein: 2g | Carbohydrates: 3g | Fat: 0g
Saturated Fat: 0g | Cholesterol: 1mg | Sodium: 32mg | Fiber: 0g | PCF Ratio: 39-56-5 | Exchange Approx.:
1 Low-Fat Milk for entire pot of soup; divide accordingly per serving

INGREDIENTS | SERVES 4

Any previous condensed soup recipe
1 cup skim milk (or soy milk or water)

To use any of the homemade condensed soup recipes as soup, add 1 cup of skim milk (or soy milk or water) to a pan. Stir using a spoon or whisk to blend. Cook over medium heat for 10 minutes until mixture begins to simmer.

Season according to taste.

Chicken and Mushroom Rice Casserole

PER SERVING: Calories: 165 | Protein: 9g | Carbohydrates: 30g | Fat: 1g | Saturated Fat: 0g | Cholesterol: 15mg
Sodium: 41mg | Fiber: 3g | PCF Ratio: 23-71-6 | Exchange Approx.: 1 Very Lean Meat, 1 Starch, 1 Vegetable

INGREDIENTS | SERVES 8

1 recipe Condensed Cream of Chicken Soup (page 122)

1 cup diced chicken breast

1 large onion, chopped

½ cup chopped celery

1 cup uncooked rice (not instant rice)

Freshly ground black pepper, to taste (optional)

1 teaspoon dried Herbes de Provence blend (Appendix C), optional

2 cups boiling water

2½ cups chopped broccoli flowerets

1 cup sliced fresh mushrooms

1. Preheat oven to 350°F. In 4-quart casserole dish (large enough to prevent boilovers in oven) treated with nonstick spray, combine condensed soup, chicken breast, onion, celery, rice, and seasonings; mix well. Pour boiling water over top; bake, covered, 30 minutes.

2. Stir casserole; add broccoli and mushrooms. Replace cover; return to oven to bake additional 20–30 minutes, or until celery is tender and rice has absorbed all liquid.

Main Dish Pork and Beans

PER SERVING: Calories: 153 | Protein: 11g | Carbohydrates: 24g | Fat: 2g | Saturated Fat: 1g
Cholesterol: 18mg | Sodium: 146mg | Fiber: 5g | PCF Ratio: 29-61-10 | Exchange Approx.:
2 Lean Meats, ½ Fruit/Misc. Carbohydrate

INGREDIENTS | SERVES 4

1⅓ cups cooked pinto beans

2 tablespoons ketchup

¼ teaspoon Dijon mustard

¼ teaspoon dry mustard

1 teaspoon cider vinegar

4 tablespoons diced red onion

1 tablespoon 100% maple syrup

1 teaspoon brown sugar

¼ pound (4 ounces) slow-cooked shredded pork

⅛ cup (2 tablespoons) apple juice or cider

Preheat oven to 350°F. In casserole dish treated with nonstick spray, combine beans, ketchup, Dijon mustard, dry mustard, vinegar, onion, syrup, and brown sugar. Layer meat over top of bean mixture. Pour apple juice or cider over pork. Bake 20–30 minutes, or until mixture is well heated and bubbling. Stir well before serving.

Easy Oven Beef Burgundy

PER SERVING: Calories: 266 | Protein: 34g | Carbohydrates: 12g | Fat: 6g | Saturated Fat: 2g | Cholesterol: 82mg
Sodium: 388mg | Fiber: 2g | PCF Ratio: 56-20-23 | Exchange Approx.: 4 Lean Meats, 2 Vegetables, 1 Fat

INGREDIENTS | SERVES 4

2 tablespoons all purpose flour
1 pound beef round, cubed
1 cup carrots, sliced
1 cup onions, chopped
1 cup celery, sliced
1 clove garlic, finely chopped
¼ teaspoon pepper
¼ teaspoon marjoram
¼ teaspoon thyme
½ teaspoon salt
2 tablespoons balsamic vinegar
½ cup dry red wine
½ cup water
1 cup fresh mushrooms, sliced

1. Preheat oven to 325°F.

2. Dredge meat cubes in flour; place in 3-quart covered baking dish or dutch oven. Add carrots, onions, celery, garlic, pepper, marjoram, thyme, salt, and vinegar; combine.

3. Pour red wine and water over mixture. Cover and bake 1 hour.

4. Remove from oven; mix in mushrooms.

5. Return to oven for 1 hour, or until beef cubes are tender.

Eggplant and Tomato Stew

PER SERVING: Calories: 135 | Protein: 4g | Carbohydrates: 26g | Fat: 3g | Saturated Fat: 1g | Cholesterol: 0mg
Sodium: 22mg | Fiber: 9g | PCF Ratio: 12-69-19 | Exchange Approx.: ½ Fat, 4 Vegetables

INGREDIENTS | SERVES 4

2 eggplants, trimmed but left whole
2 teaspoons olive oil
1 medium-sized Spanish onion, chopped
1 teaspoon garlic, chopped
2 cups cooked or canned unsalted tomatoes, chopped, with liquid
Optional seasonings, to taste:
    1 teaspoon hot pepper sauce
    Ketchup
    Nonfat plain yogurt
    Fresh parsley sprigs

1. Preheat oven to 400°F.

2. Roast eggplants on baking sheet until soft, about 45 minutes. Remove all meat from eggplants.

3. In large sauté pan, heat oil; sauté onions and garlic. Add eggplant and all other ingredients, except yogurt and parsley. Remove from heat and transfer to food processor; pulse until it becomes creamy.

4. Serve at room temperature, garnished with a dollop of yogurt and parsley, if desired.

Condensed Cream of Mushroom Soup

PER RECIPE: Calories: 92 | Protein: 3g | Carbohydrates: 21g | Fat: 1g | Saturated Fat: 0g
Cholesterol: 0mg | Sodium: 13mg | Fiber: 3g | PCF Ratio: 12-84-4 | Exchange Approx.:
Will depend on serving size and preparation method

INGREDIENTS | YIELDS EQUIVALENT
OF 1 (10.75-OUNCE) CAN

½ cup water
⅛ cup Ener-G potato flour
¾ cup finely chopped fresh mushrooms
Optional ingredients:
   1 teaspoon chopped onion
   1 tablespoon chopped celery

Potato Flour Substitute?

Instant mashed potatoes can replace potato flour; however, the amount needed will vary according to the brand of potatoes. Also, you'll need to consider other factors such as added fats and hydrogenated oils.

1. In a microwave-safe covered container, microwave mushrooms (and onion and celery, if using) 2 minutes, or until tender. (About ¾ cup chopped mushrooms will yield ½ cup steamed ones.) Reserve any resulting liquid; add enough water to equal 1 cup.

2. Place all ingredients in a blender; process. The thickness of soup concentrate will vary according to how much moisture remains in mushrooms. If necessary, add 1–2 tablespoons of water to achieve a paste. (Low-sodium canned mushrooms work in this recipe, but the nutritional analysis assumes fresh mushrooms are used. Adjust sodium content accordingly.)

Traditional Stovetop Tuna-Noodle Casserole

PER SERVING: Calories: 245 | Protein: 20g | Carbohydrates: 33g | Fat: 4g | Saturated Fat: 2g | Cholesterol: 46mg | Sodium: 241mg | Fiber: 4g | PCF Ratio: 32-53-15 | Exchange Approx.: 1½ Starches, 1 Vegetable, 1 Medium-Fat Meat

INGREDIENTS | SERVES 4

1⅓ cups egg noodles (yields 2 cups when cooked)

1 recipe Condensed Cream of Mushroom Soup (page 127)

1 teaspoon steamed chopped onion

1 tablespoon steamed chopped celery

½ cup skim milk

1 ounce American, Cheddar, or Colby cheese, shredded (to yield ¼ cup)

1 cup frozen mixed peas and carrots

1 cup steamed sliced fresh mushrooms

1 can water-packed tuna, drained

1. Cook egg noodles according to package directions. Drain and return to pan.

2. Add all remaining ingredients to pan; stir to blend. Cook over medium heat, stirring occasionally, until cheese is melted. (The nutritional analysis for this recipe assumes egg noodles were cooked without salt.)

Extra-Rich Stovetop Tuna-Noodle Casserole

Add 1 medium egg (beaten) and 1 tablespoon mayonnaise to give casserole taste of rich, homemade egg noodles, while still maintaining good fat ratio. It's still less than 300 calories per serving, too! Nutritional Analysis: Calories: 275; Protein: 21g; Carbohydrates: 34g; Fat: 7g; Saturated Fat: 2g; Cholesterol: 94mg; Sodium: 281mg; Fiber: 4g; PCF Ratio: 30-48-21; Exchange Approx.: 1½ Breads, 1 Vegetable, 1 Meat, 1 Medium-Fat Meat.

Ham and Artichoke Hearts Scalloped Potatoes

PER SERVING, without salt: Calories: 269 | Protein: 21g | Carbohydrates: 31g | Fat: 8g | Saturated Fat: 4g
Cholesterol: 28mg | Sodium: 762mg | Fiber: 6g | PCF Ratio: 31-44-25 | Exchange Approx.:
1½ Lean Meats, ½ High-Fat Meat, 1½ Vegetables, 1 Starch

INGREDIENTS | SERVES 4

2 cups frozen artichoke hearts

1 cup chopped onion

4 small potatoes, thinly sliced

Sea salt and freshly ground black pepper, to taste (optional)

1 tablespoon lemon juice

1 tablespoon dry white wine

1 cup Mock Cream (page 183)

½ cup nonfat cottage cheese

1 teaspoon dried parsley

1 teaspoon garlic powder

⅛ cup freshly grated Parmesan cheese

¼ pound (4 ounces) lean ham, cubed

2 ounces Cheddar cheese, grated (to yield ½ cup)

1. Preheat oven to 300°F.

2. Thaw artichoke hearts and pat dry with a paper towel. In deep casserole dish treated with nonstick spray, layer artichokes, onion, and potatoes; lightly sprinkle salt and pepper over top (if using).

3. In a food processor or blender, combine lemon juice, wine, Mock Cream, cottage cheese, parsley, garlic powder, and Parmesan cheese; process until smooth. Pour over layered vegetables; top with ham. Cover casserole dish (with a lid or foil); bake 35–40 minutes, or until potatoes are cooked through.

4. Remove cover; top with Cheddar cheese. Return to oven another 10 minutes, or until cheese is melted and bubbly. Let rest 10 minutes before cutting.

Simple Substitutions

Artichoke hearts can be expensive. You can substitute cabbage, broccoli, or cauliflower (or a mixture of all 3) for the artichokes.

Hearty Beef Stew

PER SERVING: Calories: 326 | Protein: 26g | Carbohydrates: 32g | Fat: 10g | Saturated Fat: 3g
Cholesterol: 88mg | Sodium: 335mg | Fiber: 4g | PCF Ratio: 32-39-28 | Exchange Approx.:
3 Lean Meats, 1 Starch, 3 Vegetables

INGREDIENTS | SERVES 4

1 tablespoon olive oil

12 ounces beef round, cut into 1" cubes

1 cup onion, chopped

2 cups potatoes, cut into 1" pieces

½ cup carrots, cut into 1" pieces

1 cup green beans

½ cup turnip, peeled and cut into 1" pieces

1 tablespoon parsley

¼ teaspoon Tabasco

1 cup low-sodium V-8 Juice

¼ teaspoon salt

1 tablespoon all-purpose flour

¼ cup water

1. Heat olive oil in pressure cooker and brown meat. Add onions, potatoes, carrots, green beans, turnip, parsley, Tabasco, V-8 juice, and salt.

2. Close cover securely; place pressure regulator on vent pipe and cook 10–12 minutes with pressure regulator rocking slowly (or follow manufacturer instructions for your pressure cooker). Cool down pressure cooker at once (nonelectric pressure cookers).

3. If desired, make paste of 1 tablespoon flour and ¼ cup water; stir into stew to thicken. Heat and stir liquid until thickened.

Slow-Cook Method for Beef Stew

If you don't have a pressure cooker, you can make this in a slow cooker. First, heat olive oil in skillet. Dredge meat in 1–2 tablespoon flour; add to skillet and brown. Transfer to slow cooker; add onions, V-8, potatoes, carrots, green beans, turnip, salt, parsley, and Tabasco. Cook on low-medium 4–6 hours.

Shrimp Microwave Casserole

PER SERVING: Calories: 196 | Protein: 18g | Carbohydrates: 27g | Fat: 2g | Saturated Fat: 1g
Cholesterol: 131mg | Sodium: 290mg | Fiber: 2g | PCF Ratio: 35-56-9 | Exchange Approx.: 1 Starch,
1 Vegetable, 1 Medium-Fat Meat

INGREDIENTS | SERVES 4

1⅓ cups uncooked egg noodles (to yield 4½ [½-cup] servings)

1 cup chopped green onion

1 cup chopped green pepper

1 cup sliced mushrooms

1 recipe Condensed Cream of Celery Soup (page 122)

1 teaspoon Worcestershire sauce (see recipe for Homemade Worcestershire on page 192)

4 drops Tabasco (optional)

¼ cup diced canned pimientos

½ cup pitted, chopped ripe olives

½ cup skimmed milk

½ pound (8 ounces) cooked, deveined, shelled shrimp

1. Cook egg noodles according to package directions; drain and keep warm.

2. Place green onion and green pepper in covered microwave-safe dish; microwave on high 1 minute. Add mushrooms; microwave another minute, or until all vegetables are tender.

3. Add soup, Worcestershire sauce, Tabasco (if using), pimiento, olives, and milk; stir well. Microwave, covered, 1–2 minutes, until mixture is hot and bubbly.

4. Add cooked shrimp and noodles; stir to mix. Microwave 30 seconds to 1 minute, or until mixture is hot.

CHAPTER 9

Pasta, Rice, Grains, and Beans

Tuscan Pasta Fagioli

PER SERVING: Calories: 317 | Protein: 15g | Carbohydrates: 54g | Fat: 6g | Saturated Fat: 1g | Cholesterol: 2mg
Sodium: 248mg | Fiber: 11g | PCF Ratio: 18-65-17 | Exchange Approx.: 3 Starches, ½ Vegetable, 1 Fat

INGREDIENTS | SERVES 6

2 tablespoons olive oil

⅓ cup onion, chopped

3 cloves garlic, minced

½ pound tomatoes, peeled and chopped

5 cups low-sodium vegetable stock

¼ teaspoon freshly ground pepper

3 cups cannellini beans, rinsed and drained

2½ cups whole-grain pasta shells

2 tablespoons Parmesan cheese

1. Heat olive oil in large pot; gently cook onions and garlic until soft but not browned. Add tomatoes, vegetable stock, and pepper.

2. Purée 1½ cups of cannellini beans in food processor or blender; add to stock. Cover and simmer 20–30 minutes.

3. While stock is simmering, cook pasta until al dente; drain. Add remaining beans and pasta to stock; heat through. Serve with Parmesan cheese.

Brown Rice and Vegetable Sauté

PER SERVING: Calories: 154 | Protein: 5g | Carbohydrates: 26g | Fat: 4g | Saturated Fat: 1g | Cholesterol: 0mg
Sodium: 352mg | Fiber: 3g | PCF Ratio: 12-64-24 | Exchange Approx.: 1 Starch, 1½ Vegetables, 1 Fat

INGREDIENTS | SERVES 4

½ cup brown rice

1 cup water

1 tablespoon olive oil

½ cup onions, chopped

1 cup red bell peppers, chopped

1 teaspoon garlic, minced

4 ounces mushrooms, sliced

12-ounce package fresh bean sprouts

1 tablespoon reduced-sodium soy sauce

1 teaspoon fresh ginger, grated

1. Add rice to water, bring to boil. Reduce heat; cover and simmer 35–40 minutes, until cooked.

2. In large nonstick skillet or wok, heat olive oil. Add onions, red pepper, and garlic; cook until onion is translucent.

3. Add mushrooms, bean sprouts, and soy sauce; cook on low heat 3 minutes.

4. Add rice and ginger; mix ingredients. Cook on low additional 2–3 minutes.

Squash and Bulgur Pilaf

PER SERVING: Calories: 151 | Protein: 5g | Carbohydrates: 22g | Fat: 6g | Saturated Fat: 1g | Cholesterol: 0mg
Sodium: 190mg | Fiber: 5g | PCF Ratio: 13-54-32 | Exchange Approx.: 1 Starch, ½ Vegetable, 2 Fats

INGREDIENTS | SERVES 6

1 tablespoon olive oil

½ cup onions, chopped

1 teaspoon garlic, minced

1½ cups yellow summer squash, cut into ½" pieces

1 cup bulgur wheat

1 tablespoon olive oil

2 cups low-sodium chicken broth

½ teaspoon cinnamon

¼ cup dried currants

¼ cup walnuts, chopped

1. In large nonstick skillet, sauté onions, garlic, yellow squash, and bulgur wheat in olive oil until onions are tender, about 5 minutes.

2. Stir in chicken broth and cinnamon; heat to boiling. Reduce heat and simmer, covered, 10 minutes.

3. Stir in currants; continue to simmer additional 15 minutes. Add walnuts just before serving.

Herbed Quinoa with Sundried Tomatoes

PER SERVING: Calories: 119 | Protein: 5g | Carbohydrates: 21g | Fat: 2g | Saturated Fat: 0g | Cholesterol: 0mg
Sodium: 193mg | Fiber: 2g | PCF Ratio: 17-71-12 | Exchange Approx.: 1 Starch, ½ Very-Lean Meat, 2 Fat

INGREDIENTS | SERVES 6

½ tablespoon olive oil

¼ cup onion, chopped

1 clove garlic, minced

1 cup quinoa

2 cups low-sodium chicken broth

½ cup fresh mushrooms, sliced

6 sundried tomatoes, cut into ¼" pieces

1 teaspoon Italian-blend seasoning

1. In medium saucepan, heat olive oil; sauté onions and garlic.

2. Rinse quinoa in very fine mesh strainer before cooking. Add quinoa and broth to saucepan; bring to a boil for 2 minutes. Add mushrooms, sundried tomatoes, and Italian seasoning.

3. Reduce heat and cover. Cook 15 minutes, or until all water is absorbed.

Cooking Time for Quinoa

Quinoa takes no longer to cook than rice or pasta, usually about 15 minutes. You can tell quinoa is cooked when grains have turned from white to transparent and spiral-like germ has separated from seed.

Whole-Grain Noodles with Caraway Cabbage

PER SERVING: Calories: 169 | Protein: 6g | Carbohydrates: 27g | Fat: 5g | Saturated Fat: 1g | Cholesterol: 0mg
Sodium: 250mg | Fiber: 5g | PCF Ratio: 14-60-26 | Exchange Approx.: 1 Starch, 1 Vegetable, 1 Fat

INGREDIENTS | SERVES 6

2 tablespoons olive oil
½ cup onion, chopped
2 cups cabbage, coarsely chopped
1½ cups Brussels sprouts, trimmed and halved
2 teaspoons caraway seed
1½ cups low-sodium chicken broth
¼ teaspoon fresh ground pepper
¼ teaspoon salt
6 ounces whole-grain noodles

1. Heat olive oil in large saucepan; sauté onions for about 5 minutes until translucent.

2. Add cabbage and Brussels sprouts; cook over medium heat 3 minutes.

3. Stir in caraway seed, broth, pepper, and salt; Cover and simmer 5–8 minutes, until vegetables are crisp-tender.

4. Cook noodles in boiling water until tender; drain.

5. Mix noodles and vegetables together in a large bowl; serve.

Bleu Cheese Pasta

PER SERVING: Calories: 213 | Protein: 12g | Carbohydrates: 21g | Fat: 9g | Saturated Fat: 4g | Cholesterol: 17mg
Sodium: 317mg | Fiber: 1g | PCF Ratio: 23-39-37 | Exchange Approx.: ½ High-Fat Meat, ½ Very-Lean Meat,
½ Lean Meat, 1 Starch, ½ Fat

INGREDIENTS | SERVES 4

2 teaspoons olive oil
1 clove garlic, minced
½ cup nonfat cottage cheese
2 ounces crumbled bleu cheese
Skim milk as needed (optional)
2 cups cooked pasta
¼ cup freshly grated Parmesan cheese
Freshly ground black pepper (optional)

1. Heat olive oil in large nonstick skillet. Add garlic; sauté 1 minute. Lower heat; stir in cottage cheese and cook for 2 minutes.

2. Add bleu cheese; stir to combine. Thin sauce with a little skim milk, if necessary.

3. Add pasta; toss with sauce. Divide into 4 equal servings; serve immediately, topped with freshly ground pepper, if desired.

Red and White Bean Salad

PER SERVING: Calories: 86 | Protein: 8g | Carbohydrates: 27g | Fat: 6g | Saturated Fat: 1g | Cholesterol: 0mg
Sodium: 7mg | Fiber: 7g | PCF Ratio: 17-55-27 | Exchange Approx.: 1½ Starches, 1 Vegetable,
½ Very-Lean Meat, 2 Fats

INGREDIENTS | SERVES 8

2 cups navy beans, cooked

2 cups red beans, cooked

1 cup arugula, chopped

¼ cup lemon juice

3 tablespoons olive oil

¼ teaspoon fresh ground pepper

1 cup red onion, thinly sliced

8 ounces cherry tomatoes, cut in half

1. Combine beans together in medium bowl.

2. Whisk together arugula, lemon juice, olive oil, and pepper; pour over beans.

3. Add onions; toss lightly to mix. Let mixture refrigerate at least 3 hours.

4. Just before serving, toss in cherry tomatoes; mix lightly.

About Arugula

Arugula has several other names such as rocket, rugula, roquette, and rucola. It is sometimes found in baby greens or mesclun mixes. It has a nutty and peppery flavor, which can add interest to a salad or sandwich. Give arugula a try!

Quick Tomato Sauce

PER SERVING, without salt: Calories: 40 | Protein: 1g | Carbohydrates: 6g | Fat: 2g | Saturated Fat: 0g
Cholesterol: 0mg | Sodium: 10mg | Fiber: 1g | PCF Ratio: 9-49-42 | Exchange Approx.: 1 Vegetable, ½ Fat

INGREDIENTS | SERVES 8

2 pounds very ripe tomatoes

2 tablespoons extra-virgin olive oil

2 cloves garlic, minced

½ teaspoon ground cumin

2 large sprigs fresh thyme, or ½ teaspoon dried thyme

1 bay leaf

Kosher or sea salt and freshly ground black pepper, to taste (optional)

3 tablespoons total of chopped fresh basil, oregano, tarragon, and parsley or cilantro, or a combination of all the listed herbs, to taste. If using dried herbs, reduce the amount to 1 tablespoon

1. Peel and seed tomatoes; chop with knife or food processor.

2. Heat large skillet; add olive oil. Reduce heat to low; sauté garlic and cumin.

3. Add tomatoes, thyme, bay leaf, salt, and pepper, if using. If using dried herbs, add now. Simmer, uncovered, over medium heat 8–10 minutes, stirring often; reduce heat to maintain a simmer, if necessary. Simmer until tomatoes are soft and sauce has thickened, about 30 minutes. Discard bay leaf and thyme sprigs; adjust seasoning to taste. If using fresh herbs, add just before serving.

Fresh Garden Tomato Sauce

PER SERVING: Calories: 154 | Protein: 6g | Carbohydrates: 26g | Fat: 5g | Saturated Fat: 1g | Cholesterol: 0mg
Sodium: 867mg | Fiber: 6g | PCF Ratio: 15-61-25 | Exchange Approx.: 5 Vegetables, 1 Fat

INGREDIENTS | SERVES 12

3 tablespoons olive oil

1 cup celery, chopped

1 cup onion, finely chopped

1 cup green (or sweet red) pepper, chopped

2 cloves garlic, crushed

8 cups fresh tomatoes, peeled and crushed

1 (5½-ounce) can tomato paste

1 cup zucchini, grated

1 tablespoon fresh oregano, chopped

1 tablespoon fresh basil, chopped

½ teaspoon crushed red pepper

½ cup dry red wine

1. In large, heavy sauce pan or Dutch oven, heat oil. Add celery, onion, and peppers; sauté 5 minutes. Add crushed garlic; sauté additional 2 minutes.

2. Add crushed tomatoes, tomato paste, zucchini, oregano, basil, and red pepper. Bring to a boil; reduce heat and simmer 2–3 hours.

3. Add wine during last 30 minutes of cooking.

Basic Tomato Sauce

PER SERVING, without salt: Calories: 37 | Protein: 1g | Carbohydrates: 5g | Fat: 2g | Saturated Fat: 0g
Cholesterol: 0mg | Sodium: 9mg | Fiber: 1g | PCF Ratio: 9-55-36 | Exchange Approx.: 1½ Vegetables

INGREDIENTS | YIELDS ABOUT 5 CUPS; SERVING SIZE: ¼ CUP

2 tablespoons olive oil

2 cups coarsely chopped yellow onion

½ cup sliced carrots

2 cloves garlic, minced

4 cups canned Italian plum tomatoes with juice

1 teaspoon dried oregano

1 teaspoon dried basil

¼ teaspoon sugar

Kosher or sea salt and freshly ground black pepper, to taste (optional)

Dash of ground anise seed (optional)

1. Heat olive oil in large, deep skillet or saucepan over medium-high heat. Add onions, carrots, and garlic; sauté until onions are transparent. (For a richer-tasting sauce, allow onions to caramelize or reach a light golden brown.)

2. Purée tomatoes in food processor.

3. Add the puréed tomatoes, oregano, basil, and sugar to onion mixture along with salt, pepper, and anise, if using. Simmer, partially covered, 45 minutes.

4. If you prefer a smoother sauce, process sauce in food processor again.

Culinary Antacids

Stir in 2 teaspoons Smucker's Low-Sugar Grape Jelly to tame hot chili or acidic sauces such as tomato sauce. You won't really notice the flavor of the jelly, and it will do a great job of reducing any tart, bitter, or acidic tastes in your sauce.

Fusion Lo Mein

PER SERVING: Calories: 126 | Protein: 5g | Carbohydrates: 26g | Fat: 1g | Saturated Fat: 0g | Cholesterol: 0mg
Sodium: 35mg | Fiber: 4g | PCF Ratio: 14-77-9 | Exchange Approx.: 1 Starch, 1 Vegetable, ½ Fruit

INGREDIENTS | SERVES 6

2 tablespoons rice vinegar

2 tablespoons thawed pineapple-orange juice

2 teaspoons minced shallots

2 teaspoons lemon juice

1 teaspoon cornstarch

1 teaspoon Worcestershire sauce (see recipe for homemade on page 192)

1 teaspoon honey

2 cloves garlic, minced

1 teaspoon olive oil

¾ cup chopped green onions

1 cup diagonally sliced (¼" thick) carrots

1 cup julienned yellow bell pepper

1 cup julienned red bell pepper

3 cups small broccoli florets

1 cup fresh bean sprouts

1½ cups cooked pasta

1. In food processor or blender, combine vinegar, juice concentrate, shallots, lemon juice, cornstarch, Worcestershire, honey, and garlic; process until smooth.

2. Heat wok or large nonstick skillet coated with cooking spray over medium-high heat until hot; add olive oil. Add onions; stir-fry 1 minute.

3. Add carrots, bell peppers, and broccoli; stir-fry another minute. Cover pan; cook 2 more minutes.

4. Add vinegar mixture and sprouts. Bring mixture to a boil; cook, uncovered, 30 seconds, stirring constantly.

5. Add cooked pasta; toss to mix.

Roasted Butternut Squash Pasta

PER SERVING: Calories: 216 | Protein: 5g | Carbohydrates: 40g | Fat: 5g | Saturated Fat: 1g | Cholesterol: 0mg
Sodium: 8mg | Fiber: 2g | PCF Ratio: 9-70-21 | Exchange Approx.: 2 Starches, 1 Fat, ½ Vegetable

INGREDIENTS | SERVES 4

1 butternut squash
4 teaspoons extra-virgin olive oil
1 clove garlic, minced
1 cup chopped red onion
2 teaspoons red wine vinegar
¼ teaspoon dried oregano
2 cups cooked pasta
Freshly ground black pepper (optional)

Tip

For added flavor, use roasted instead of raw garlic. Roasting garlic causes it to caramelize, adding a natural sweetness.

1. Preheat oven to 400°F. Cut squash in half and scoop out seeds. Using nonstick spray, coat 1 side of 2 pieces of heavy-duty foil large enough to wrap squash halves. Wrap squash in foil; place on a baking sheet. Bake 1 hour, or until tender.

2. Scoop out baked squash flesh and discard rind; rough-chop. Add olive oil, garlic, and onion to nonstick skillet; sauté for about 5 minutes until onion is transparent. (Alternatively, put oil, garlic, and onion in covered microwave-safe dish; microwave on high 2–3 minutes.)

3. Remove pan from heat; stir in vinegar and oregano. Add squash; stir to coat in onion mixture. Add pasta; toss to mix. Season with freshly ground black pepper, if desired.

Pasta with Creamed Clam Sauce

PER SERVING: Calories: 226 | Protein: 15g | Carbohydrates: 24g | Fat: 7g | Saturated Fat: 2g | Cholesterol: 25mg
Sodium: 209mg | Fiber: 1g | PCF Ratio: 27-43-30 | Exchange Approx.: 1 Lean Meat, 1 Starch, 1 Fat, ½ Skim Milk

INGREDIENTS | SERVES 4

1 (6½-ounce) can chopped clams

4 teaspoons olive oil

1 clove garlic, minced

1 tablespoon dry white wine or dry vermouth

½ cup Mock Cream (page 183)

¼ cup freshly grated Parmesan cheese

2 cups cooked pasta

Freshly ground black pepper, to taste (optional)

1. Drain clams; reserve juice. Heat olive oil in large nonstick skillet. Add garlic; sauté 1 minute; stir in clams and sauté another minute. With slotted spoon, transfer clams to a bowl; cover to keep warm.

2. Add wine and reserved clam juice to skillet; bring to a boil and reduce by half. Lower heat and add Mock Cream; cook for about 2–3 minutes, being careful not to boil cream.

3. Stir in Parmesan cheese; continue to heat another minute, stirring constantly.

4. Toss sauce with pasta; divide into 4 equal servings. Top each serving with a tablespoon of Parmesan cheese and freshly ground black pepper, if desired.

Pasta with Artichokes

PER SERVING: Calories: 308 | Protein: 10g | Carbohydrates: 47g | Fat: 9g | Saturated Fat: 2g
Cholesterol: 2mg | Sodium: 87mg | Fiber: 3g | PCF Ratio: 13-60-27 | Exchange Approx.:
1 Medium-Fat Meat, 2 Vegetables, 1 Starch, 2 Fats

INGREDIENTS | SERVES 4

1 (10-ounce) package frozen artichoke hearts

1¼ cups water

1 tablespoon lemon juice

4 teaspoons olive oil

2 cloves garlic, minced

¼ cup sundried tomatoes packed in oil, drained and chopped

¼ teaspoon red pepper flakes

2 teaspoons dried parsley

2 cups cooked pasta

¼ cup grated Parmesan cheese

Freshly ground black pepper, to taste (optional)

1. Cook artichokes in water and lemon juice according to package directions; drain, reserving ¼ cup of liquid. Cool artichokes; cut into quarters.

2. Heat olive oil in nonstick skillet over medium heat. Add garlic; sauté 1 minute. Reduce heat to low. Stir in artichokes and tomatoes; simmer 1 minute. Stir in reserved artichoke liquid, red pepper, and parsley; simmer 5 minutes.

3. Pour artichoke sauce over pasta in a large bowl; toss gently to coat. Sprinkle with cheese and top with pepper, if desired.

Tip

You can decrease amount of water to 3 tablespoons and add with artichokes and lemon juice to covered microwave-safe dish. Microwave according to package directions; reserve all liquid. This results in stronger lemon flavor, which compensates for lack of salt in recipe.

Quinoa with Roasted Vegetables

**PER SERVING: Calories: 120 | Protein: 4g | Carbohydrates: 9g | Fat: 4g | Saturated Fat: 0g | Cholesterol: 0mg
Sodium: 151mg | Fiber: 4g | PCF Ratio: 12-62-26 | Exchange Approx.: 1 Starch, 1 Vegetable, 2 Fats**

INGREDIENTS | SERVES 4

⅔ cup green pepper

½ cup red pepper (mildly hot variety)

3 cups eggplant, cut into 1" cubes

2 cloves garlic, finely chopped

1 tablespoon olive oil

½ teaspoon Texas Seasoning (Appendix C)

¼ teaspoon cumin

½ cup quinoa

1 cup water

¼ teaspoon salt

Another Idea

Cook quinoa as outlined in steps 3 and combine with 3 cups of Oven-Roasted Ratatouille recipe found on page 155. Nutritional analysis for 1 cup serving: Calories: 162; Protein: 7g; Carbohydrates: 26g; Fat: 3g; Saturated Fat: 0g; Cholesterol: 1mg; Sodium: 202mg; Fiber: 4g; PCF Ratio: 13-69-18; Exchange Approx.: 1 Starch, 2 Vegetables, ½ Fat.

1. Preheat oven to 375°F. Combine peppers, eggplant, garlic, olive oil, Texas seasoning, and cumin in 2-quart baking dish. Cover and roast 20 minutes.

2. Remove cover; continue to roast in oven for about 30 minutes until vegetables are browned and cooked soft. Remove from oven; replace cover.

3. Rinse quinoa in very fine mesh strainer before cooking. Bring water and salt to a boil; add quinoa and bring to a boil for 5 minutes. Cover; remove from heat and let stand 15 minutes.

4. Once quinoa is cooked and all water is absorbed, add roasted vegetables and serve.

Kasha-Stuffed Red Peppers

PER SERVING: Calories: 383 | Protein: 22g | Carbohydrates: 54g | Fat: 12g | Saturated Fat: 5g
Cholesterol: 40mg | Sodium: 387mg | Fiber: 11g | PCF Ratio: 22-53-25 | Exchange Approx.:
2 Starches, 4 Vegetables, 1½ Lean Meats, 2 Fats

INGREDIENTS | SERVES 4

2 pounds red peppers (4 large)
1 cup kasha
1 egg white, lightly beaten
Nonstick cooking spray
2 cups low-sodium beef broth
4 ounces lean ground beef
1 cup onion, finely chopped
5 ounces (½ package) frozen chopped spinach, thawed and drained
½ cup feta cheese, crumbled
½ cup canned diced tomatoes
1 teaspoon oregano
⅛ teaspoon crushed red pepper
1½ cups water

Save the Tomato Juice

Most canned tomatoes are packed in juice or puréed tomato. When you open a can, save juices and add to recipes when liquids are called for. In this recipe, tomato juice from a can could substitute for some water used to cook peppers in.

1. Remove tops of red peppers and remove seeds; set aside.

2. Mix kasha and egg white together in small bowl. In large nonstick saucepan sprayed with nonstick cooking spray, add kasha; cook over high heat 2–3 minutes, stirring constantly, until kasha kernels are separated.

3. Add beef broth slowly. Reduce heat; cover and cook 7–10 minutes, until kasha kernels are tender. Transfer to large bowl.

4. Brown beef in small nonstick skillet. Add onions; cook 2–3 minutes, until slightly softened.

5. Add beef mixture and chopped spinach to cooked kasha; mix well. Stir in feta cheese, diced tomato, oregano, and crushed red pepper. Divide mixture equally; stuff each red pepper. Place peppers in 9" × 9" baking dish.

6. Pour water around peppers. Cover with foil; bake in 375°F oven 60–75 minutes, or until peppers are cooked.

Whole-Wheat Couscous Salad

PER SERVING: Calories: 153 | Protein: 4g | Carbohydrates: 15g | Fat: 9g | Saturated Fat: 1g | Cholesterol: 0mg
Sodium: 85mg | Fiber: 2g | PCF Ratio: 9-38-52 | Exchange Approx.: 1 Starch, 2 Fats

INGREDIENTS | SERVES 8

1 cup low-sodium chicken broth

¼ cup dried currants

½ teaspoon cumin

¾ cup whole-wheat couscous

¼ cup olive oil

2 tablespoons lemon juice

1 cup broccoli, chopped and steamed to crisp-tender

3 tablespoons pine nuts

1 tablespoon fresh parsley, chopped

1. Combine chicken broth, currants, and cumin; bring to a boil. Remove from heat; stir in couscous. Cover and let sit until cool. Fluff couscous with fork 2–3 times during the cooling process.

2. Whisk together olive oil and lemon juice.

3. Add steamed broccoli and pine nuts to couscous. Pour oil and lemon juice over couscous; toss lightly. Garnish with chopped parsley.

Aren't Currants Just Small Raisins?

Dried currants may look like miniature raisins, but they are actually quite different. Currants are berries from a shrub, not a vine, and there are red and black varieties. Black currants are rich in phytonutrients and antioxidants. They have twice the potassium of bananas and four times the vitamin C of oranges!

Pasta with Tuna Alfredo Sauce

PER SERVING: Calories: 278 | Protein: 33g | Carbohydrates: 21g | Fat: 5g | Saturated Fat: 2g | Cholesterol: 32mg
Sodium: 401mg | Fiber: 1g | PCF Ratio: 50-31-18 | Exchange Approx.: 1½ Very-Lean Meats, 1½ Lean Meats,
1½ Carbohydrates/Starches

INGREDIENTS | SERVES 4

1 cup nonfat cottage cheese

1 tablespoon skim milk

2 teaspoons olive oil

1 clove garlic, minced

2 (6-ounce) cans tuna packed in water, drained

⅛ cup (2 tablespoons) dry white wine

¼ cup freshly grated Parmesan cheese

2 cups cooked pasta

Freshly ground black pepper, to taste (optional)

1. Process cottage cheese and skim milk in food processor or blender until smooth. Set aside.

2. Heat olive oil in large nonstick skillet. Add garlic; sauté 1 minute. Stir in tuna; sauté another minute.

3. Add wine to skillet; bring to a boil. Lower heat; add cottage cheese mixture. Cook for about 5 minutes, being careful not to let it boil.

4. Stir in Parmesan; continue to heat 1 minute, stirring constantly.

5. Add pasta; toss with sauce. Divide into 4 equal servings; serve immediately, topped with freshly ground pepper, if desired.

CHAPTER 10

Vegetables

Oven-Baked Red Potatoes

PER SERVING: Calories: 120 | Protein: 2g | Carbohydrates: 26g | Fat: 1g | Saturated Fat: 0g
Cholesterol: 0g | Sodium: 587mg | Fiber: 2g | PCF Ratio: 7-84-9 | Exchange Approx.: 1 Starch

INGREDIENTS | SERVES 4

1 pound (16 ounces) small red potatoes, halved

¼ cup fresh lemon juice

1 teaspoon olive oil

1 teaspoon sea salt

¼ teaspoon freshly ground pepper

Preheat oven to 350°F. Arrange potatoes in 13" × 9" ovenproof casserole dish. Combine remaining ingredients; pour over potatoes. Bake 30–40 minutes, or until potatoes are tender, turning 3–4 times to baste.

Remember the Roasting "Rack"

Use caution when roasting potatoes with meat: Potatoes will act like a sponge, soaking up fat. Your best option is to use lean cuts of meat and elevate them and vegetables above fat by putting them on a roasting rack in the pan or making a "bridge" with the celery to elevate the meat. Discard celery when done.

Healthy Onion Rings

PER SERVING, without salt: Calories: 111 | Protein: 4g | Carbohydrates: 22g | Fat: 1g | Saturated Fat: 0g
Cholesterol: 1mg | Sodium: 255mg | Fiber: 1g | PCF Ratio: 16-80-4 | Exchange Approx.: 1 Vegetable, 1 Starch

INGREDIENTS | SERVES 4

1 cup yellow onion slices (¼" thick)

½ cup flour

½ cup nonfat plain yogurt

½ cup bread crumbs

Sea salt and freshly ground black pepper, to taste (optional)

1. Preheat oven to 350°F. Dredge onion slices in flour; shake off any excess. Dip onions in yogurt; dredge through bread crumbs.

2. Prepare baking sheet with nonstick cooking spray. Arrange onion rings on pan; bake 15–20 minutes. Place under broiler additional 2 minutes to brown. Season with salt and pepper, if desired.

Sweet Potato Crisps

PER SERVING, without salt: Calories: 89 | Protein: 1g | Carbohydrates: 16g | Fat: 2g | Saturated Fat: 1g
Cholesterol: 0mg | Sodium: 7mg | Fiber: 9g | PCF Ratio: 6-70-24 | Exchange Approx.: 1 Starch, ½ Fat

INGREDIENTS | SERVES 2

1 small sweet potato or yam
1 teaspoon olive oil
Sea salt and freshly ground black pepper, to taste (optional)

1. Preheat oven to 400°F. Scrub sweet potato and pierce flesh several times with fork. Place on microwave-safe plate; microwave 5 minutes on high. Remove from microwave; wrap in aluminum foil. Set aside 5 minutes.

2. Remove foil; peel and cut into French fries. Spread on baking sheet treated with nonstick spray; spritz with olive oil. Bake 10–15 minutes, or until crisp. There's a risk that sweet potato strips will caramelize and burn; check often while cooking to ensure this doesn't occur. Lower oven temperature, if necessary. Season with salt and pepper, if desired.

Sweet Potatoes with Onions and Apple

PER SERVING: Calories: 127 | Protein: 2g | Carbohydrates: 28g | Fat: 1g | Saturated Fat: 0g
Cholesterol: 1mg | Sodium: 144mg Fiber: 4g | PCF Ratio: 6-85-9 | Exchange Approx.: 1 Starch, ½ Vegetable

INGREDIENTS | SERVES 6

1 pound sweet potatoes (about 2 large)
½ teaspoon canola oil
1 cup onion, thinly sliced
1 apple, peeled and chopped
½ cup low-sodium chicken broth

1. Wash and dry sweet potatoes; pierce skins several times with fork. Microwave on high 5–8 minutes, or until tender.

2. While sweet potatoes are cooling, heat oil in large nonstick skillet over medium-high heat. Add onions; sauté until golden brown, about 10 minutes.

3. Add apple and chicken broth; cook until onions are tender and have caramelized.

4. Scoop cooked sweet potatoes from skins into microwave-safe dish; mash lightly. Cover and microwave on high 1–2 minutes, or until potatoes are heated. Top with sautéed onions and serve.

Fluffy Buttermilk Mashed Potatoes

PER SERVING, without salt: Calories: 97 | Protein: 2g | Carbohydrates: 18g | Fat: 2g | Saturated Fat: 1g
Cholesterol: 6mg | Sodium: 20mg | Fiber: 2g | PCF Ratio: 9-72-19 | Exchange Approx.: 1 Starch, ½ Fat

INGREDIENTS | SERVES 4

¾ pound (12 ounces) peeled and boiled potatoes
¼ cup warm buttermilk
2 teaspoons unsalted butter
Sea salt and freshly ground black pepper, to taste (optional)

1. Place potatoes in large bowl; partially mash.

2. Add warm buttermilk; mix well, mashing potatoes completely.

3. Stir in butter and salt and pepper, if using. If you like your mashed potatoes creamy, add some of the potato water.

French Tarragon Green Beans

PER SERVING, without salt: Calories: 59 | Protein: 0g | Carbohydrates: 5g | Fat: 3g | Saturated Fat: 1g
Cholesterol: 11mg | Sodium: 105mg | Fiber: 1g | PCF Ratio: 3-32-65 | Exchange Approx.: 1 Vegetable, 1 Fat

INGREDIENTS | SERVES 4

1½ tablespoons butter
¼ cup red onion, chopped
½ pound fresh green beans
1 tablespoon tarragon, finely chopped

1. Melt butter in nonstick pan. Add onions; sauté until translucent.

2. Add green beans. Cover and steam 2–3 minutes.

3. Add tarragon; combine well. Steam an additional 2–3 minutes.

Baked Potato Chips

PER SERVING, without salt: Calories: 119 | Protein: 2g | Carbohydrates: 18g | Fat: 5g | Saturated Fat: 1g
Cholesterol: 0mg | Sodium: 4mg | Fiber: 1g | PCF Ratio: 5-60-34 | Exchange Approx.: 1 Starch, 1 Fat

INGREDIENTS | SERVES 1

1 small white potato (3 ounces)

1 teaspoon olive oil

Sea salt and freshly ground black pepper, to taste (optional)

Tip

Nutritional Allowance for this recipe allows for teaspoon of olive oil. Even though you spritz potatoes with oil, remember chips have more surface area than fries. To cut more fat, eliminate oil (and Fat Exchange) in Baked French Fries and Baked Potato Chips by using butter-flavored or olive oil cooking spray.

1. Preheat oven to 400°F. Wash, peel, and thinly slice potato. Wrap slices in paper towel to remove any excess moisture.

2. Spread potatoes on baking sheet treated with nonstick spray; spritz with olive oil. Bake 10–15 minutes, depending on how crisp you prefer your fries. Season with salt and pepper, if your diet allows additional sodium.

Sesame Snap Peas

PER SERVING: Calories: 49 | Protein: 0g | Carbohydrates: 3g | Fat: 4g | Saturated Fat: 0g | Cholesterol: 0mg
Sodium: 149mg | Fiber: 0g | PCF Ratio: 2-27-72 | Exchange Approx.: 1 Vegetable, ½ Fat

INGREDIENTS | SERVES 4

½ tablespoon canola oil

10 ounces fresh snap peas

¼ cup scallions, thinly sliced

1 tablespoon fresh grated ginger

2 teaspoons sesame oil

1 tablespoon sesame seeds

1. Heat canola oil in large nonstick skillet or wok.

2. Add snap peas, scallions, and ginger; stir-fry until peas are crisp-tender.

3. Stir in sesame oil and sesame seeds; toss lightly and serve.

Amish-Style Turnips

PER SERVING: Calories: 80 | Protein: 2g | Carbohydrates: 12g | Fat: 3g | Saturated Fat: 2g | Cholesterol: 40mg
Sodium: 49mg | Fiber: 2g | PCF Ratio: 10-56-34 | Exchange Approx.: 1 Vegetable, ½ Starch, ½ Fat

INGREDIENTS | SERVES 6

3 cups turnips, cooked and mashed
½ cup water
1 slice whole-wheat bread
1 tablespoon butter, melted
2 tablespoons Splenda Brown Sugar Blend
½ cup low-fat milk
1 egg

1. Cook turnips in advance. If using fresh turnips, wash, peel, and cut into 1" cubes. Put in covered dish with ½ cup water; microwave on high 10–15 minutes, until tender.

2. Place bread in food processor. Using pulse setting, process until bread is consistency of fine bread crumbs.

3. In medium bowl, mix together bread crumbs, melted butter, Splenda, milk, and egg. Add cooked turnip; mix well.

4. Turn mixture into greased casserole dish. Bake uncovered in 375°F oven 30–35 minutes.

Corn Casserole

PER SERVING: Calories: 188 | Protein: 11g | Carbohydrates: 32g | Fat: 3g | Saturated Fat: 1g | Cholesterol: 10mg
Sodium: 133mg | Fiber: 2g | PCF Ratio: 23-65-13 | Exchange Approx.: 1½ Starches, 1 Skim Milk, ½ Fat

INGREDIENTS | SERVES 2

1 tablespoon finely chopped onion
1 tablespoon finely chopped green or red bell pepper
1 cup frozen or fresh corn kernels
⅛ teaspoon ground mace
Dash ground white or black pepper
¾ cup skim milk
¼ cup nonfat dry milk
1 egg
1 teaspoon butter

1. Preheat oven to 325°F. In medium-sized bowl, combine onion, bell pepper, corn, mace, and pepper; toss to mix.

2. In blender, combine milk, dry milk, egg, and butter; process until mixed. Pour over corn mixture; toss to mix.

3. Pour entire mixture into glass casserole dish treated with nonstick spray. Bake 1 hour, or until set.

Spice Side Effects

Ground mace or nutmeg can elevate blood pressure or cause an irregular heartbeat in some individuals. Check with your doctor or nutritionist before adding it to your diet.

Oven-Roasted Ratatouille

PER SERVING: Calories: 87 | Protein: 2g | Carbohydrates: 11g | Fat: 5g | Saturated Fat: 1g | Cholesterol: 0mg
Sodium: 452mg | Fiber: 3g | PCF Ratio: 9-46-46 | Exchange Approx.: 2 Vegetables, 1 Fat

INGREDIENTS | SERVES 12

5 cups eggplant, peeled and cut into ½" cubes

3 cups yellow squash, cut into ½" pieces

½ pound green beans

½ cup celery, chopped

1 cup red onion, chopped

4 cloves garlic, chopped

1 (28-ounce) can diced tomatoes

1 tablespoon fresh parsley, chopped

¼ teaspoon salt

½ teaspoon rosemary

½ teaspoon thyme

¼ cup olive oil

2 tablespoons balsamic vinegar

1. Preheat oven to 375°F. In large Dutch oven or 9" × 13" baking dish, combine eggplant, yellow squash, green beans, celery, onion, garlic, tomatoes, parsley, salt, rosemary, thyme, and olive oil.

2. Roast uncovered in oven. Stir after 30 minutes, then continue roasting another 30 minutes, or until vegetables are softened and lightly browned on top.

3. Remove from oven. Stir in balsamic vinegar and serve.

Layered Veggie Casserole

PER SERVING: Calories: 84 | Protein: 5g | Carbohydrates: 16g | Fat: 1g | Saturated Fat: 1g | Cholesterol: 3mg
Sodium: 101mg | Fiber: 4g | PCF Ratio: 20-67-13 | Exchange Approx.: 1 Vegetable, 1 Starch

INGREDIENTS | SERVES 4

1 (10-ounce) package frozen mixed vegetables

½ cup diced onion

½ cup diced green pepper

1 cup unsalted tomato juice

⅛ teaspoon celery seed

⅛ teaspoon dried basil

⅛ teaspoon dried oregano

⅛ teaspoon dried parsley

¼ teaspoon garlic powder

3 tablespoons grated Parmesan cheese, divided

1. Preheat oven to 350°F. Using large casserole dish treated with nonstick spray, layer vegetables, onion, and pepper. Mix tomato juice, seasonings, and 2 tablespoons of Parmesan; pour over vegetables. Cover and bake 1 hour.

2. Uncover; sprinkle with remaining Parmesan. Continue to bake 10 minutes, or until liquid thickens and mixture bubbles.

Season First

When readying vegetables for steaming, add fresh or dried herbs, spices, sliced or diced onions, minced garlic, grated ginger, or any other seasoning you'd normally use. Seasonings will cook into vegetables during steaming.

Baked French Fries

PER SERVING, without salt: Calories: 119 | Protein: 2g | Carbohydrates: 18g | Fat: 5g | Saturated Fat: 1g
Cholesterol: 0mg | Sodium: 4mg | Fiber: 1g | PCF Ratio: 5-60-34 | Exchange Approx.: 1 Starch, 1 Fat

INGREDIENTS | SERVES 1

1 small white potato (3 ounces)

1 teaspoon olive oil

Sea salt and freshly ground black pepper, to taste (optional)

Get a Head Start

Speed up time it takes to bake French fries! First, cook potatoes in microwave 3–4 minutes in a covered microwave-safe dish; allow to rest at least 1 minute. Dry with paper towels, if necessary; arrange on baking sheet treated with nonstick spray. Spray with flavored cooking spray or few spritzes of olive oil; bake at 400°F for 5–8 minutes to crisp.

1. Preheat oven to 400°F. Wash, peel, and slice potatoes into French fry wedges. Wrap slices in paper towel to remove any excess moisture.

2. "Oil" potatoes by placing into plastic bag with olive oil. Close bag and shake until potatoes are evenly coated. Spread on baking sheet treated with nonstick spray; bake 5–10 minutes.

3. Remove pan from oven; quickly turn potatoes. Return pan to oven; bake another 10–15 minutes, depending on how crisp you prefer your fries. Season with salt and pepper, if your diet allows additional sodium.

Crustless Zucchini and Artichoke Quiche

PER SERVING: Calories: 224 | Protein: 24g | Carbohydrates: 9g | Fat: 10g | Saturated Fat: 4g | Cholesterol: 134mg
Sodium: 798mg | Fiber: 3g | PCF Ratio: 43-16-41 | Exchange Approx.: 1 Vegetable, 1½ Lean Meats, 1½ Fats

INGREDIENTS | SERVES 4

Nonstick cooking spray

1 tablespoon olive oil

¼ cup onions, chopped

¾ cup zucchini, grated

1 cup canned artichoke hearts, cut in ½" pieces

1½ cups light Cheddar cheese, grated

2 eggs

½ cup egg whites

½ cup fat-free cottage cheese

¼ teaspoon cayenne

¼ teaspoon salt

⅛ teaspoon fresh-ground pepper

1. Preheat oven to 375°F. Spray 9" pie plate with cooking spray. In large nonstick skillet, heat olive oil; add onion and sauté until translucent.

2. Add zucchini and artichoke hearts; cook additional 3 minutes.

3. Sprinkle grated cheese in bottom of pie plate; add cooked vegetables on top of cheese.

4. In small bowl, whisk eggs, egg whites, cottage cheese, cayenne, salt, and pepper together; pour over vegetables.

5. Bake 35–40 minutes, or until set and inserted toothpick comes out clean.

Vegetable Broth

PER SERVING: Calories: 10 | Protein: 0g | Carbohydrates: 2g | Fat: 0g | Saturated Fat: 0g | Cholesterol: 0mg
Sodium: 8mg | Fiber: 1g | PCF Ratio: 11-85-4 | Exchange Approx.: 1 Free Vegetable

INGREDIENTS | YIELDS ABOUT 2½ QUARTS; SERVING SIZE: ¾ CUP

4 carrots, peeled and chopped

2 celery stalks and leaves, chopped

1 green bell pepper, seeded and chopped

2 medium zucchini, chopped

1 small onion, chopped

1 cup chopped fresh spinach

2 cups chopped leeks

½ cup chopped scallions

1 cup chopped green beans

1 cup chopped parsnips

2 bay leaves

2 cloves garlic, crushed

Sea salt and freshly ground black pepper (optional)

3 quarts water

1. Place all of ingredients in large pot; bring to a boil. Reduce heat; cover pan and simmer 30 minutes, or until vegetables are tender. Discard bay leaf.

2. Use slotted spoon to transfer vegetables to different pot; mix with some of broth for Free Exchange vegetable soup. Freeze mixture in single-serving containers to keep on hand for a quick, heat-in-the-microwave snack.

3. Strain remaining vegetables from broth; purée in blender or food processor and return to broth to add dietary fiber and body. Cool and freeze until needed.

Perpetual Broth

The easiest way to create vegetable broth is to keep a container in the freezer for saving liquid from cooked vegetables. Vegetable broth makes a great addition to sauces, soups, and many other recipes. Substitute it for meat broth in most recipes or use instead of water for cooking pasta, rice, and other grains.

Winter Vegetable Casserole

PER SERVING: Calories: 218 | Protein: 5g | Carbohydrates: 36g | Fat: 7g | Saturated Fat: 1g | Cholesterol: 18mg
Sodium: 392mg | Fiber: 5g | PCF Ratio: 9-64-27 | Exchange Approx.: 1½ Starches, 1½ Vegetables, 1 Fat

INGREDIENTS | SERVES 6

Cooking spray
1½ potatoes, thinly sliced
1½ sweet potatoes, thinly sliced
1 cup parsnips, peeled and sliced
1 cup turnips, sliced
½ cup onions, chopped
3 tablespoons butter
3 tablespoons all-purpose flour
½ teaspoon salt
¼ teaspoon white pepper
1½ cups low-fat milk

1. Spray 2-quart casserole dish with cooking spray.

2. Clean, peel, and slice potatoes, sweet potatoes, parsnips, and turnips; combine. Chop onions and set aside.

3. In small saucepan, melt butter; add flour, salt, and pepper to make a roux. Gradually stir in milk, cooking over low heat; stir well with wire whisk.

4. Bring milk to a boil, stirring constantly, until milk has thickened into a sauce, about 10 minutes. Remove from heat.

5. Arrange ½ of sliced vegetables in casserole dish; top with ½ of chopped onion and white sauce; repeat to make second layer. Cover and cook at 350°F for 45 minutes. Uncover and continue to cook until all vegetables are tender, about 60–70 minutes.

6. Let casserole stand 10 minutes before serving.

Broccoli Raab with Pine Nuts

PER SERVING: Calories: 110 | Protein: 5g | Carbohydrates: 6g | Fat: 8g | Saturated Fat: 1g | Cholesterol: 0mg
Sodium: 229mg | Fiber: 4g | PCF Ratio: 18-20-62 | Exchange Approx.: 1 Vegetable, 1 Fat

INGREDIENTS | SERVES 4

¾ pound broccoli raab, cooked

1 tablespoon olive oil

4 cloves garlic, chopped

¼ cup sundried tomatoes, chopped

2 tablespoons pine nuts

¼ teaspoon salt

¼ teaspoon crushed red pepper

Preventing Bitter Broccoli Raab

Broccoli raab and other leafy greens (mustard or collard greens) can have a bitter taste once cooked. Rather than add extra salt to offset bitterness, this recipe calls for blanching 2 minutes, which helps reduce bitterness. Blanching should be done as quickly as possible by starting with water at full rolling boil, then removing after 2 minutes of boiling. If allowed to cook too long, the boiling process will reduce the amount of water-soluble nutrients found in the vegetables.

1. Prepare and blanch broccoli before beginning recipe: Rinse well and trim stems. Loosely chop leafy parts, then blanch in 2 quarts boiling water 2 minutes. Drain well.

2. Heat olive oil in large skillet; add garlic. Sauté garlic 1–2 minutes; add cooked broccoli. Toss garlic and broccoli together well, so that oil and garlic are mixed evenly.

3. Add remaining ingredients; cook additional 2–3 minutes, until broccoli is tender.

Roasted-Garlic Mashed Potatoes

PER SERVING, without salt: Calories: 126 | Protein: 4g | Carbohydrates: 23g | Fat: 2g
Saturated Fat: 1g | Cholesterol: 6 mg | Sodium: 31mg | Fiber: 3g | PCF Ratio: 13-70-17
Exchange Approx.: 1 Starch, 1 Vegetable, ½ Fat

INGREDIENTS | SERVES 4

4 cloves roasted garlic (see Dry-Roasted Garlic on page 26)

1 small onion, chopped

¾ pound (12 ounces) peeled, cooked potatoes

2 cups cauliflower, steamed and drained

¼ cup buttermilk

⅛ cup nonfat cottage cheese

2 teaspoons unsalted butter

Sea salt and freshly ground black pepper, to taste (optional)

Combine all ingredients; whip until fluffy. If potatoes or cauliflower are overly moist, add buttermilk gradually until whipped mixture reaches desired consistency. Combining steamed cauliflower with the potatoes allows you to increase the portion size without significantly changing the flavor of the mashed potatoes.

Gravy Substitute

Instead of using gravy, sprinkle crumbled bleu cheese or grated Parmesan over mashed potatoes. Just remember that cheese is a Meat Exchange and adjust approximations accordingly.

Spaghetti Squash and Vegetable Mix

PER SERVING: Calories: 127 | Protein: 4g | Carbohydrates: 16g | Fat: 6g | Saturated Fat: 3g | Cholesterol: 5mg
Sodium: 169mg | Fiber: 2g | PCF Ratio: 12-47-41 | Exchange Approx.: 1 Starch, 1 Fat

INGREDIENTS | SERVES 6

2 pounds spaghetti squash
Cooking spray
1 cup peas, fresh or frozen
2 tablespoons butter
8 ounces cherry tomatoes, cut in half
1 ounce grated Romano cheese
¼ teaspoon fresh ground pepper

Pasta Alternative

Spaghetti squash is a wonderful alternative to pasta because it is packed with vitamins, minerals, and fiber. While it has a consistency similar to spaghetti, it is much lower in carbohydrates: 1 cup of cooked spaghetti squash has 15 grams of carbohydrate, while 1 cup of cooked spaghetti has approximately 45 grams!

1. Cut spaghetti squash in half and scoop out seeds. Spray 9" × 13" baking dish with cooking spray; place squash halves face down. Bake at 400°F for 45 minutes, or until squash is soft-cooked.

2. When squash is cool enough to handle, use a fork to scoop out cooked squash from the outer shell. Scoop into a medium-sized microwaveable bowl.

3. In separate small saucepan, lightly steam peas 2–3 minutes. Add to squash, along with butter; mix well.

4. Place covered bowl in microwave; cook on high 2–3 minutes.

5. Add cherry tomato halves and top with Romano cheese and pepper before serving.

Greens in Garlic with Pasta

PER SERVING, without salt: Calories: 176 | Protein: 8g | Carbohydrates: 26g | Fat: 5g | Saturated Fat: 1g
Cholesterol: 0mg | Sodium: 17mg | Fiber: 3g | PCF Ratio: 17-58-25 | Exchange Approx.: 1 Free
Vegetable, 1 Fat, 1 Starch, ½ Lean Meat

INGREDIENTS | SERVES 4

2 teaspoons olive oil

4 cloves garlic, crushed

6 cups, tightly packed loose-leaf greens (baby mustard, turnip, chard)

2 cups cooked pasta

2 teaspoons extra-virgin olive oil

¼ cup freshly grated Parmesan cheese

Salt and freshly ground black pepper, to taste (optional)

1. Place sauté pan over medium heat. When hot, add 2 teaspoons of olive oil and garlic. Cook, stirring frequently, until golden brown, 3–5 minutes, being careful not to burn garlic, as that makes it bitter.

2. Add greens; sauté until coated in garlic oil. Remove from heat.

3. In large serving bowl, add pasta, cooked greens, 2 teaspoons of extra-virgin olive oil, and Parmesan cheese; toss to mix. Serve immediately, and season as desired.

Sweet or Salty?

In most cases, when you add a pinch (less than ⅛ teaspoon) of sugar to a recipe, you can reduce the amount of salt without noticing a difference. Sugar acts as a flavor enhancer and magnifies the effect of the salt.

Vegetable Frittata

PER SERVING: Calories: 171 | Protein: 12g | Carbohydrates: 11g | Fat: 9g | Saturated Fat: 4g | Cholesterol: 195mg
Sodium: 252mg | Fiber: 2g | PCF Ratio: 28-24-48 | Exchange Approx.: 1 Vegetable, 1 Lean Meat, 2½ Fats

INGREDIENTS | SERVES 4

1½ tablespoons olive oil

4 ounces red pepper, chopped

3 large eggs

4 ounces egg substitute (or egg whites)

4 ounces asparagus, cut diagonally in 1" pieces

¾ cup potatoes, cooked and cubed

⅓ cup feta cheese, crumbled

1 teaspoon oregano

1. Preheat oven to 350°F. Using ovenproof nonstick skillet, heat olive oil over medium heat. Add red peppers; cook until softened.

2. In medium bowl, beat together eggs and egg substitute. Add asparagus, potatoes, feta, and oregano.

3. Pour eggs into skillet; gently stir until eggs on bottom of pan begin to set. Gently pull cooked eggs from side of skillet, allowing liquid uncooked egg on top to come in contact with heated skillet. Repeat, working all around skillet, until most of eggs on top have begun to set.

4. Transfer skillet to oven; bake until top is set and dry to the touch, about 3–5 minutes. Loosen frittata around edges of skillet and invert onto serving plate.

Gnocchi

PER SERVING: Calories: 139 | Protein: 4g | Carbohydrates: 28g | Fat: 1g | Saturated Fat: 0g
Cholesterol: 23mg | Sodium: 9mg | Fiber: 1g | PCF Ratio: 12-82-6 | Exchange Approx.: 1½ Starches

INGREDIENTS | SERVES 8

1 cup boiled and mashed potatoes

2 cups all-purpose or semolina flour

1 egg

Old-Country Secrets

Italian cooks sometimes toss each helping of gnocchi in a teaspoon of melted butter and sugar, then sprinkle it with cinnamon to serve it as a dessert. This adds 1 Fat exchange and 1 Carbohydrate exchange to the recipe.

1. Combine potatoes, flour, and egg in large bowl; knead until dough forms a ball. Finished dough should be smooth, pliable, and slightly sticky.

2. Shape 4 equal portions of dough into long ropes, about ¾" in diameter. On floured surface, cut ropes into ½" pieces. Press thumb or forefinger into each piece to create an indentation. (Some gnocchi chefs also like to roll each piece with a fork to add a distinctive texture.)

3. Bring large pot of water to a boil. Drop in gnocchi, being careful amount you add doesn't stop water from boiling. Cook 3–5 minutes, or until gnocchi rise to top. Remove from water with slotted spoon. Serve immediately, or, if you make it in batches, put finished gnocchi on a platter to be set in a warm oven.

CHAPTER 11

Salads

Cucumbers with Minted Yogurt

PER SERVING: Calories: 31 | Protein: 2g | Carbohydrates: 4g | Fat: 1g | Saturated Fat: 0g | Cholesterol: 2mg
Sodium: 52mg | Fiber: 1g | PCF Ratio: 27-56-17 | Exchange Approx.: 1 Vegetable

INGREDIENTS | SERVES 8

1 cup nonfat plain yogurt

1 clove garlic, finely chopped

¼ teaspoon cumin

1 teaspoon lemon zest

½ cup mint

1 tablespoon lemon juice

¼ teaspoon salt

4 cups cucumbers, seeded and chopped

1. Combine yogurt, garlic, cumin, lemon zest, mint, lemon juice, and salt in blender or food processor; blend until smooth.

2. Add yogurt mixture to cucumbers; mix. Chill before serving.

Orange-Avocado Slaw

PER SERVING, without salt: Calories: 60 | Protein: 2g | Carbohydrates: 5g | Fat: 5g | Saturated Fat: 1g
Cholesterol: 0mg | Sodium: 14mg | Fiber: 2g | PCF Ratio: 11-27-62 | Exchange Approx.: 1 Fat, ½ Free Vegetable

INGREDIENTS | SERVES 10

¼ cup orange juice

½ teaspoon curry powder

⅛ teaspoon ground cumin

¼ teaspoon sugar

1 teaspoon white wine vinegar

1 tablespoon olive oil

1 avocado, peeled and chopped

5 cups broccoli slaw mix

Sea salt and freshly ground black pepper, to taste (optional)

1. In bowl, whisk together orange juice, curry powder, cumin, sugar, and vinegar. Add oil in stream, whisking until emulsified.

2. In large bowl, toss avocado with slaw mix; drizzle with vinaigrette. Chill until ready to serve. Season with salt and pepper, if desired.

Minted Lentil and Tomato Salad

PER SERVING: Calories: 136 | Protein: 4g | Carbohydrates: 11g | Fat: 9g | Saturated Fat: 1g | Cholesterol: 0mg
Sodium: 211mg | Fiber: 4g | PCF Ratio: 10-31-59 | Exchange Approx.: ½ Starch, 1 Vegetable, ½ Lean Meat, 2 Fats

INGREDIENTS | SERVES 6

1 cup dry lentils

2 cups water

½ cup onion, chopped

2 teaspoons garlic, minced

¼ cup celery, chopped

½ cup green pepper, chopped

½ cup parsley, finely chopped

2 tablespoons fresh mint, finely chopped, or 2 teaspoons dried

¼ cup lemon juice

¼ cup olive oil

½ teaspoon salt

1 cup fresh tomato, diced

1. Place lentils and water in medium-sized saucepan; bring to a quick boil. Reduce heat; cover and cook on low 15–20 minutes, or until tender. Drain and transfer to medium bowl.

2. Add onion, garlic, celery, green pepper, parsley, and mint; mix well.

3. In small bowl, whisk together lemon juice, olive oil, and salt. Pour into lentils; mix well. Cover and refrigerate several hours.

4. Before serving, mix in diced tomatoes.

Tomato and Cucumber Salad with Mint

PER SERVING: Calories: 68 | Protein: 1g | Carbohydrates: 7g | Fat: 5g | Saturated Fat: 1g | Cholesterol: 0mg
Sodium: 202mg | Fiber: 1g | PCF Ratio: 5-32-63 | Exchange Approx.: 1 Vegetable, 1 Fat

INGREDIENTS | SERVES 6

2 cucumbers

⅓ cup red wine vinegar

1 teaspoon sugar

½ teaspoon salt

2 cups tomatoes, chopped

⅔ cup red onion, chopped

¼ cup fresh mint, chopped

2 tablespoons olive oil

1. Cut cucumbers in ½" wide pieces; place in medium bowl.

2. Add vinegar, sugar, and salt; stir. Let stand at room temperature for 15 minutes.

3. Add tomatoes, red onion, mint, and olive oil; toss lightly to blend.

Broccoli-Cauliflower Slaw

PER SERVING: Calories: 117 | Protein: 6g | Carbohydrates: 13g | Fat: 5g | Saturated Fat: 1g | Cholesterol: 0mg
Sodium: 46mg | Fiber: 1g | PCF Ratio: 19-42-39 | Exchange Approx.: 1 Misc. Carbohydrate, 1 Fat

INGREDIENTS | SERVES 8

4 cups raw broccoli flowerets

4 cups raw cauliflower

½ cup real mayonnaise

1 cup cottage cheese, 1% fat

3 tablespoons tarragon vinegar

1 tablespoon balsamic vinegar

⅛ cup packed brown sugar

3 tablespoons red onion

1. Put broccoli and cauliflower in food processor; pulse-process to consistency of shredded cabbage. Pour into a bowl.

2. Place remaining ingredients in food processor; process until smooth. Pour resulting dressing over broccoli-cauliflower mixture; stir. Chill until ready to serve.

Tip

Substituting cottage cheese for some mayonnaise cuts fat and calories considerably. Cut them even more by using nonfat cottage cheese and mayonnaise.

Marinated Roasted Peppers and Eggplant

PER SERVING: Calories: 179 | Protein: 2g | Carbohydrates: 14g | Fat: 14g | Saturated Fat: 2g | Cholesterol: 0mg
Sodium: 5mg | Fiber: 6g | PCF Ratio: 5-29-66 | Exchange Approx.: 3 Vegetables, 3 Fats

INGREDIENTS | SERVES 4

1 pound sweet red peppers

1 large eggplant, sliced into ¼" thick rounds

2 tablespoons olive oil

1 tablespoon balsamic vinegar

2 tablespoons olive oil

1 tablespoon onion, finely chopped

1 teaspoon oregano

Fresh ground pepper

1. Follow procedure for roasting red peppers on page 196. Set aside.

2. Brush eggplant slices with 2 tablespoons olive oil; place on grill. Grill on both sides for about 5 minutes each until softened. Remove from grill and place in container. Add roasted peppers to container.

3. Prepare marinade by whisking together balsamic vinegar, 2 tablespoons olive oil, chopped onion, oregano, and pepper; pour over vegetables. Cover and refrigerate.

Spinach Salad with Pomegranate

PER SERVING: Calories: 107 | Protein: 4g | Carbohydrates: 8g | Fat: 8g | Saturated Fat: 1g | Cholesterol: 0mg
Sodium: 259mg | Fiber: 3g | PCF Ratio: 13-26-61 | Exchange Approx.: 1 Vegetable, 2 Fats

INGREDIENTS | SERVES 6

1 pound fresh spinach
½ cup red onion, very thinly sliced
8 ounces fresh tomatoes, cut into ½"
wedges
⅓ cup walnuts, chopped
½ teaspoon salt
¼ cup lemon juice
1½ tablespoons olive oil
¼ cup pomegranate seeds

1. Wash spinach thoroughly and drain well; loosely chop.

2. Add onions, tomato, and walnuts; toss lightly.

3. In small bowl, whisk together salt, lemon juice, and olive oil. Drizzle over salad; toss lightly.

4. Garnish salad with pomegranate seeds.

Tabbouleh

PER SERVING: Calories: 144 | Protein: 3g | Carbohydrates: 15g | Fat: 9g | Saturated Fat: 1g | Cholesterol: 0mg
Sodium: 212mg | Fiber: 4g | PCF Ratio: 7-38-55 | Exchange Approx.: ½ Starch, 1 Vegetable, 2 Fats

INGREDIENTS | SERVES 6

1 cup boiling water
½ cup bulgur wheat
1 cup fresh parsley, packed and finely chopped
⅓ cup fresh mint, finely chopped
½ cup red onion, finely chopped
1 cup cucumber, chopped
¼ cup lemon juice
¼ cup olive oil
½ teaspoon salt
Fresh-ground pepper, to taste
1 cup fresh tomato, chopped
2 cups leaf lettuce (optional)

1. In small bowl, pour boiling water over bulgur wheat; let stand 20 minutes.

2. When bulgur is softened, drain and squeeze out any excess water using a colander lined with cheesecloth.

3. Combine parsley, mint, onion, cucumber, and wheat. Add lemon juice, olive oil, salt, and ground pepper; mix well.

4. Cover and refrigerate at least 3 hours.

5. Just before serving, add chopped tomatoes; toss lightly. Serve as is or on bed of leaf lettuce.

Tomatoes Stuffed with Quinoa Salad

PER SERVING: Calories: 180 | Protein: 5g | Carbohydrates: 24g | Fat: 9g | Saturated Fat: 2g | Cholesterol: 4mg
Sodium: 78mg | Fiber: 4g | PCF Ratio: 11-49-40 | Exchange Approx.: ½ Starch, 2½ Vegetables, 2½ Fats

INGREDIENTS | SERVES 6

½ cup quinoa

1 cup water

6 large (3 pounds) tomatoes

1½ cups cucumber, peeled and finely diced

⅓ cup fresh parsley, chopped

¼ cup fresh mint, chopped

½ cup red onion, finely chopped

3 tablespoons feta cheese, crumbled

2 tablespoons lemon juice

3 tablespoons olive oil

1. Rinse quinoa in fine mesh strainer before cooking. To cook: Place quinoa and water in small saucepan; bring to a boil. Reduce heat; cover and cook until all water is absorbed, about 15 minutes. Cool.

2. Prepare tomatoes: remove caps and hollow out, leaving shell about ½" thick.

3. In mixing bowl, combine quinoa, cucumbers, parsley, mint, red onion, and feta cheese.

4. Mix lemon juice and olive oil together; pour over quinoa and vegetables.

5. Stuff tomatoes with mixture and serve.

Wilted Lettuce with a Healthier Difference

PER SERVING: Calories: 71 | Protein: 2g | Carbohydrates: 7g | Fat: 5g | Saturated Fat: 1g | Cholesterol: 0mg
Sodium: 9mg | Fiber: 2g | PCF Ratio: 8-34-57 | Exchange Approx.: 2 Free Vegetables, 1 Fat

INGREDIENTS | SERVES 1

½ teaspoon olive oil

¼ cup chopped red onion

1½ cups tightly packed loose-leaf lettuce

¼ teaspoon lemon juice or your choice of vinegar

½ teaspoon extra-virgin olive oil, walnut oil, or almond oil

Optional seasonings to taste:

    Dried herbs of your choice, such as thyme or parsley

    Pinch of sugar

    Pinch of toasted sesame seeds or grated Parmesan cheese

1. In heated nonstick skillet treated with nonstick spray, add ½ teaspoon of olive oil and all red onion. Sauté until onion is almost transparent; add greens. Sauté greens until warmed and wilted.

2. In salad bowl, whisk lemon juice with ½ teaspoon oil. Add pinch of herbs and sugar, if using; whisk into oil mixture. Add wilted greens; toss with dressing. Top salad with pinch of toasted sesame seeds or Parmesan cheese, if desired. Serve immediately.

Taco Salad

PER SERVING: Calories: 426 | Protein: 23g | Carbohydrates: 58g | Fat: 13g | Saturated Fat: 7g
Cholesterol: 30mg | Sodium: 380mg | Fiber: 13g | PCF Ratio: 21-53-26 | Exchange Approx.:
1 Lean Meat, 1 High-Fat Meat, 3 Starches, 2 Vegetables

INGREDIENTS | SERVES 8

1 recipe Vegetable and Bean Chili (see page 38)

8 cups tightly packed salad greens

8 ounces Cheddar cheese, shredded (to yield 2 cups)

8 ounces nonfat corn chips

Nonstarchy free-exchange vegetables of your choice, such as chopped celery, onion, or banana or jalapeño peppers (optional)

1. Prepare Vegetable and Bean Chili.

2. Divide salad greens between 8 large bowls. Top with chili, Cheddar cheese, corn chips, and vegetables or peppers, if using.

Green Bean and Mushroom Salad

PER SERVING: Calories: 131 | Protein: 2g | Carbohydrates: 9g | Fat: 10g | Saturated Fat: 1g | Cholesterol: 0mg
Sodium: 4mg | Fiber: 3g | PCF Ratio: 7-26-67 | Exchange Approx.: 2 Fats, 2 Vegetables

INGREDIENTS | SERVES 4

2 cups fresh small green beans, ends trimmed

1½ cups sliced fresh mushrooms

½ cup chopped red onion

3 tablespoons extra-virgin olive, canola, or corn oil

1 tablespoon balsamic or red wine vinegar

1 clove garlic, minced

½ teaspoon sea salt (optional)

¼ teaspoon freshly ground pepper (optional)

1. Cook green beans in large pot of unsalted boiling water for 5 minutes. Drain in colander; immediately plunge into bowl of ice water to stop cooking process and retain bright green color of the beans.

2. Once beans are cool, drain and place in large bowl. If you'll be serving salad immediately, add mushrooms and onions to bowl; toss to mix. (Otherwise, as recommended earlier, chill beans separately and add to salad immediately before serving.)

3. To make dressing, combine oil and vinegar in small bowl. Whisk together with garlic; pour over salad. Toss lightly; season with salt and pepper, if desired. Serve immediately.

Spinach Salad with Apple-Avocado Dressing

PER SERVING: Calories: 122 | Protein: 2g | Carbohydrates: 8g | Fat: 10g | Saturated Fat: 1g | Cholesterol: 0mg
Sodium: 90mg | Fiber: 3g | PCF Ratio: 7-25-68 | Exchange Approx.: 2½ Fats, 1 Free Vegetable

INGREDIENTS | SERVES 4

¼ cup unsweetened apple juice

1 teaspoon (or up to 1 tablespoon) cider vinegar

1 clove garlic, minced

1 teaspoon Bragg's Liquid Aminos or soy sauce

½ teaspoon Worcestershire sauce (see recipe for homemade on page 192)

2 teaspoons olive oil

1 avocado, peeled and chopped

2½ cups tightly packed spinach and other salad greens

½ cup thinly sliced red onion

½ cup sliced radishes

½ cup bean sprouts

1. In blender or food processor, combine juice, vinegar (the amount of which will depend on how you like your dressing), garlic, Liquid Aminos, Worcestershire, oil, and avocado; process until smooth.

2. In large bowl, toss greens, onions, radishes, and bean sprouts. Pour dressing over salad; toss again.

Greek Pasta Salad

PER SERVING: Calories: 420 | Protein: 12g | Carbohydrates: 31g | Fat: 29g | Saturated Fat: 5g | Cholesterol: 13mg
Sodium: 312mg | Fiber: 6g | PCF Ratio: 11-28-61 | Exchange Approx.: 1 Medium-Fat Meat, 1 Meat Substitute,
1 Free Vegetable, 1½ Starches, 4 Fats

INGREDIENTS | SERVES 4

1 tablespoon lemon juice

3 tablespoons olive oil

1 teaspoon dried oregano

1 teaspoon Dijon mustard

1 clove garlic, minced

2 cups cooked pasta

1 cup slivered blanched almonds

1 cup sliced cucumber

1 cup diced fresh tomato

½ cup chopped red onion

½ cup Greek olives

2 ounces crumbled feta cheese

1½ cups romaine lettuce leaves

1. In large salad bowl, whisk lemon juice with olive oil, oregano, mustard, and garlic. Cover and refrigerate 1 hour or up to 12 hours.

2. Immediately before serving, toss pasta with almonds, cucumbers, tomatoes, onions, olives, and feta cheese. Serve over lettuce.

Sweet and Savory Side Salad

For 1 serving of easy, versatile salad or simple dressing over salad greens, mix ¾ cup shredded carrots, ¼ cup diced celery, 1 tablespoon raisins, and 1 teaspoon frozen pineapple juice concentrate. Nutritional analysis: Calories: 31.00; Protein: 0.47g; Carbohydrates: 64g; Fat: 0.07g; Saturated Fat: 0.01g; Cholesterol: 0.00mg; Sodium: 141mg; Fiber: 1.00g; PCF Ratio: 6-92-2; Exchange Approx.: ½ Fruit, 1 Free Vegetable, 1 Vegetable.

Mandarin Snap Pea Salad

PER SERVING, without dressing: | Calories: 76 | Protein: 4g | Carbohydrates: 16g | Fat: 0g | Saturated Fat: 0g
Cholesterol: 0mg | Sodium: 344mg | Fiber: 4g | PCF Ratio: 19-78-3 | Exchange Approx.: ½ Starch,
1 Vegetable, ½ Lean Meat, ½ Fat

INGREDIENTS | SERVES 8

¾ pound snap peas, cut into ½" pieces

1 cup canned mandarin oranges, drained

1½ cups canned kidney beans, rinsed
and drained

1 cup red onion, thinly sliced

½ cup fresh parsley, chopped

2 cups cabbage, chopped

⅓ cup poppy seed dressing (recipe
below)

1. In medium bowl, combine snap peas, mandarin oranges, kidney beans, onions, parsley, and cabbage.

2. Mix in poppy seed dressing; refrigerate several hours before serving.

Poppy Seed Dressing

Combine ½ cup red wine vinegar, ¼ cup orange juice, 3 tablespoons lemon juice, ½ cup canola oil, 1 teaspoon Splenda Brown Sugar Blend, 1 teaspoon dry mustard, 1 teaspoon salt, and 1 tablespoon poppy seeds; mix well in covered jar. Store in refrigerator. Nutritional analysis 1 ounce serving (1½ tablespoons): 68 Calories; Protein: 0g; Carbohydrates: 9g; Fat: 7g; Saturated Fat: 1g; Cholesterol: 0mg; Sodium: 148mg; PCF Ration: 1-9-90; Exchange Approx.: 1½ Fats

Zesty Feta and Olive Salad

PER SERVING: Calories: 109 | Protein: 3g | Carbohydrates: 6g | Fat: 8g | Saturated Fat: 3g
Cholesterol: 132mg | Sodium: 326mg | Fiber: 2g | PCF Ratio: 11-22-66 | Exchange Approx.: 1 Vegetable, 2 Fats

INGREDIENTS | SERVES 4

2 ounces crumbled feta

1 small red onion, diced

½ cup chopped celery

½ cup diced cucumber

1 clove garlic, minced

1 teaspoon lemon zest

1 teaspoon orange zest

1 cup halved very small cherry tomatoes

½ cup mix of green and kalamata olives, pitted and sliced

1 tablespoon extra-virgin olive oil

2 tablespoons minced fresh Italian parsley

2 teaspoons minced fresh oregano

1 teaspoon minced fresh mint

1 tablespoon minced fresh cilantro (optional)

Large romaine or butter lettuce leaves

Freshly ground black pepper

1. In a large bowl, place feta, onion, celery, cucumber, garlic, lemon zest, orange zest, tomatoes, and olives; mix.

2. Add olive oil and fresh herbs; toss again.

3. Arrange lettuce leaves on 4 salad plates; spoon feta salad on top. Top with pepper and serve.

Avocado and Peach Salad

PER SERVING, without salt: | Calories: 160 | Protein: 2g | Carbohydrates: 15g | Fat: 11g
Saturated Fat: 2g | Cholesterol: 0mg | Sodium: 11mg | Fiber: 4g | PCF Ratio: 6-35-59
Exchange Approx.: 3 Fats, 1 Free Vegetable, ½ Fruit

INGREDIENTS | SERVES 4

⅛ cup water

⅛ cup frozen orange juice concentrate

1 clove garlic, crushed

1 teaspoon rice wine vinegar

1 tablespoon extra-virgin olive oil

½ teaspoon vanilla

1½ cups tightly packed baby arugula

2 tablespoons tarragon leaves

1 avocado, peeled and diced

1 peach, peeled and diced

½ cup thinly sliced Vidalia onion

Kosher or sea salt and freshly ground
black pepper, to taste (optional)

1. In measuring cup, whisk water, orange juice concentrate, garlic, vinegar, oil, and vanilla together until well mixed.

2. Prepare salad by arranging layers of arugula and tarragon, then avocado, peach, and onions, then drizzle with prepared orange juice vinaigrette. Season with salt and pepper, if desired, and serve.

Experiment Sensibly

When it comes to new herbs and spices, err on the side of caution. Not sure whether or not you like a seasoning? Mix all other ingredients together and test a bite of salad with pinch of herb or spice before adding it to the entire recipe.

Honey Dijon Tuna Salad

PER SERVING: Calories: 194 | Protein: 22g | Carbohydrates: 24g | Fat: 1g | Saturated Fat: 0g
Cholesterol: 0mg | Sodium: 575mg | Fiber: 4g | PCF Ratio: 45-49-6 | Exchange Approx.:
1 Lean Meat, 2 Vegetables, ½ Fruit, ½ Skim Milk

INGREDIENTS | SERVES 1

¼ cup canned tuna in water, drained

½ cup diced celery

¼ cup diced onion

¼ cup seeded and diced red or green pepper

4 ounces (½ small container) nonfat plain yogurt

1 teaspoon Dijon mustard

1 teaspoon lemon juice

¼ teaspoon honey

1 tablespoon raisins

1 cup tightly packed iceberg lettuce or other salad greens

1. Use fork to flake tuna into bowl. Add all other ingredients except lettuce; mix well. Serve on lettuce or greens.

2. Alternate serving suggestion: Mix with ½ cup chilled, cooked pasta before dressing salad greens. Adds 1 Starch Exchange choice.

Golden Raisin Smoked Turkey Salad

PER SERVING: Calories: 355 | Protein: 21g | Carbohydrates: 62g | Fat: 8g | Saturated Fat: 2g
Cholesterol: 19mg | Sodium: 723mg | Fiber: 4g | PCF Ratio: 21-61-18 | Exchange Approx.:
1 Very-Lean Meat, 1 Lean Meat, 1½ Vegetables, 3 Fats, 1 Fruit, 1 Misc. Carbohydrate

INGREDIENTS | YIELDS 4 GENEROUS-SIZED SALADS

4 cups chopped broccoli

2 cups chopped cauliflower

3 shallots, chopped

1⅓ cups golden raisins

1 cup 1% cottage cheese

¼ cup real mayonnaise

¼ cup firm silken tofu

3 tablespoons tarragon vinegar

1 tablespoon balsamic vinegar

¼ cup brown sugar

¼ pound (4 ounces) smoked turkey breast, chopped

Freshly ground pepper (optional)

4 cups salad greens

1. Combine broccoli, cauliflower, and shallots in large bowl; stir in raisins.

2. In blender or food processor, mix together cottage cheese, mayonnaise, tofu, vinegars, and brown sugar until smooth.

3. Toss dressing over broccoli, cauliflower, raisins, shallots, and turkey. Season with freshly ground pepper to taste. Chill until ready to serve, over salad greens.

Tip

Because of the smoked turkey, this salad is high in sodium. If you're on a sodium-restricted diet, substitute regular cooked turkey or chicken breast. Punch up the flavor by adding 1 teaspoon Bragg's Liquid Aminos or Homemade Worcestershire Sauce (see page 192).

Rainbow Potato Salad

PER SERVING: Calories: 146 | Protein: 5g | Carbohydrates: 29g | Fat: 2g | Saturated Fat: 0g
Cholesterol: 0mg | Sodium: 615mg | Fiber: 5g | PCF Ratio: 12-77-11 | Exchange Approx.: 1½ Starches

INGREDIENTS | SERVES 6

2 pounds red potatoes (6 medium)

⅓ cup carrots, finely chopped

¼ cup onion, finely chopped

¼ cup green pepper, finely chopped

¼ cup yellow or red bell pepper, finely chopped

2 tablespoons red wine vinegar

2 tablespoons lemon juice

¼ teaspoon celery seed

1 teaspoon sugar

½ teaspoon salt

2 tablespoons light mayonnaise

1. Wash and scrub red potatoes. Place whole potatoes in pot and cover with water. Boil over medium heat for about 20 minutes until potatoes are cooked. Drain; set aside to cool.

2. Combine carrots, onion, peppers, vinegar, lemon juice, celery seed, sugar, and salt in small bowl; mix. Cover and refrigerate for 2–3 hours.

3. After vegetables have marinated, add light mayonnaise; mix well.

4. Cut potatoes (with skins on) into ½" cubes.

5. In large bowl, combine potatoes and vegetables; mix well.

Potato and Snow Pea Salad

PER SERVING: Calories: 139 | Protein: 5g | Carbohydrates: 28g | Fat: 1g | Saturated Fat: 0g | Cholesterol: 3mg
Sodium: 223mg | Fiber: 3g | PCF Ratio: 13-78-9 | Exchange Approx.: 1 Starch, 1 Vegetable, ½ Fat

INGREDIENTS | SERVES 8

2 pounds red potatoes (6 medium)
3 slices bacon
½ cup onion, chopped
¾ pound snow peas, cut in ½" pieces
½ teaspoon salt
¼ cup apple cider vinegar

1. Wash and scrub red potatoes. Place whole potatoes in pot; cover with water. Boil over medium heat for 20 minutes until potatoes are cooked. Drain and chill. Once chilled, cut into ½" cubes.

2. Cut bacon slices into ½" pieces. Place in nonstick fry pan with onions; fry for 3–4 minutes until crisp. There should be a light coating of fat in pan from bacon. If there is excess fat, pour off before going to Step 3.

3. Add snow peas; toss with bacon and onion mixture for 2 minutes. Remove from heat.

4. Dissolve salt into cider vinegar; mix into snow peas.

5. In large bowl, combine potatoes and snow peas; mix well.

Summer Salad

PER SERVING: Calories: 73 | Protein: 2g | Carbohydrates: 7g | Fat: 5g | Saturated Fat: 1g | Cholesterol: 0mg
Sodium: 109mg | Fiber: 2g | PCF Ratio: 9-36-55 | Exchange Approx.: 1½ Vegetables, 1 Fat

INGREDIENTS | SERVES 6

2 cups snap peas, cut into 1" pieces

2 cups summer squash, cut into ½" pieces

½ cup carrots, chopped

3 tablespoons mushrooms, minced

2 cups cucumbers, chopped

¼ cup onion, thinly sliced

2 tablespoons canola oil

2 tablespoons balsamic vinegar

¼ teaspoon salt

¼ teaspoon thyme

¼ teaspoon marjoram

1. Combine snap peas, squash, carrots, and mushrooms; steam for 2–3 minutes, until crisp-tender. Cool and refrigerate.

2. When cooled, add cucumbers and onions.

3. Whisk together canola oil, balsamic vinegar, salt, thyme, and marjoram. Pour over vegetables; toss lightly. Serve.

Tip

Add the oil and vinegar dressing just before serving. Minimize the exposure of vinegar to certain vegetables such as snap peas or green beans to retain their bright colors.

CHAPTER 12

Salad Dressings, Salsas, and Sauces

Creamy Feta Vinaigrette

PER SERVING: Calories: 31 | Protein: 1g | Carbohydrates: 1g | Fat: 2g | Saturated Fat: 1g
Cholesterol: 4mg | Sodium: 57mg | Fiber: 0g | PCF Ratio: 17-17-66 | Exchange Approx.: ½ Fat

INGREDIENTS | **YIELDS ABOUT ⅔ CUP; SERVING SIZE: 1 TABLESPOON**

½ cup plain low-fat yogurt

1 tablespoon lemon juice

1 tablespoon olive oil

1½ ounces feta cheese

2 teaspoons mint

½ packet Splenda (optional)

Fresh-ground pepper, to taste

Process all ingredients in food processor or blender. Chill before serving.

Raspberry Tarragon Vinaigrette

PER SERVING: Calories: 120 | Protein: 0g | Carbohydrates: 9g | Fat: 9g | Saturated Fat: 1g
Cholesterol: 0mg | Sodium: 0mg | Fiber: 0g | PCF Ratio: 0-33-67 | Exchange Approx.: 2 Fats

INGREDIENTS | **YIELDS ¾ CUP; SERVING SIZE: 1 TABLESPOON**

½ cup olive oil

¼ cup raspberry vinegar (see recipe at right)

2 teaspoons lemon juice

½ tablespoon tarragon, finely chopped

Salt and pepper, to taste

Combine ingredients in a covered jar; shake thoroughly.

Making Raspberry Vinegar

Combine 2 cups raspberries, lightly mashed; 2 tablespoons honey; and 2 cups red wine vinegar in nonstick saucepan. Simmer uncovered for 10 minutes; cool. Place in 1-quart jar; store at room temperature for 3 weeks. Strain vinegar from berries; pour strained vinegar into an empty wine bottle. Cork or cap.

Buttermilk Dressing

PER SERVING, without salt: Calories: 14 | Protein: 1g | Carbohydrates: 3g | Fat: 0g | Saturated Fat: 0g
Cholesterol: 0mg | Sodium: 18mg | Fiber: 0g | PCF Ratio: 25-71-5 | Exchange Approx.: 1 Free

INGREDIENTS | YIELDS ABOUT ⅔ CUP; SERVING SIZE: 1 TABLESPOON

½ cup plain nonfat yogurt
1 tablespoon buttermilk powder
1 teaspoon prepared mustard
¼ teaspoon cider vinegar
1 tablespoon light brown sugar
¼ teaspoon paprika
⅛ teaspoon hot red pepper (optional)
¼ teaspoon salt (optional)

Place all ingredients in jar; put lid on and shake vigorously until mixed. Refrigerate any unused portions. May be kept in refrigerator up to 3 days.

Mock Cream

PER RECIPE: Calories: 147 | Protein: 14g | Carbohydrates: 21g | Fat: 1g | Saturated Fat: 1g
Cholesterol: 8mg | Sodium: 221mg | Fiber: 0g | PCF Ratio: 39-57-3 | Exchange Approx.: 1½ Skim Milks

INGREDIENTS | YIELDS 1¼ CUPS; SERVING SIZE: 2 TABLESPOONS

1 cup skim milk
¼ cup nonfat dry milk

Process ingredients in blender until mixed. Use as a substitute for heavy cream.

Comparative Analysis

Using 1¼ cups heavy cream would give you the following breakdown: Calories: 5102; Protein: 6g; Carbohydrates: 17g; Fat: 527g; Saturated Fat: 340g; Cholesterol: 2079mg; Sodium: 516mg; Fiber: 0g; PCF Ratio: 2-3-95; Exchange Approx.: 11 Fats.

Bleu Cheese Dressing

PER SERVING: Calories: 24 | Protein: 1g | Carbohydrates: 1g | Fat: 2g | Saturated Fat: 1g
Cholesterol: 3mg | Sodium: 52mg | Fiber: 0g | PCF Ratio: 21-23-57 | Exchange Approx.: ½ Fat

INGREDIENTS | YIELDS 6 TABLESPOONS;
SERVING SIZE: 1
TABLESPOON

2 tablespoons Plain non-fat yogurt
1 tablespoon cottage cheese
1 tablespoon real mayonnaise
½ teaspoon lemon juice
½ teaspoon honey
1 tablespoon plus 2 teaspoons crumbled
bleu cheese

Put yogurt, cottage cheese, mayonnaise, lemon juice, and honey in blender; process until smooth. Fold in bleu cheese.

Dijon Vinaigrette

PER SERVING: Calories: 74 | Protein: 0g | Carbohydrates: 1g | Fat: 8g | Saturated Fat: 1g
Cholesterol: 0mg | Sodium: 266mg | Fiber: 0g | PCF Ratio: 1-2-97 | Exchange Approx.: 2 Fats

INGREDIENTS | YIELDS ABOUT 5
TABLESPOONS;
SERVING SIZE: 1
TABLESPOON

1 tablespoon Dijon mustard
½ teaspoon sea salt
½ teaspoon freshly ground black pepper
1 tablespoon red wine vinegar
3 tablespoons virgin olive oil

Put all ingredients in small bowl; use wire whisk or fork to mix.

The Vinegar-Oil Balancing Act
The easiest way to tame too much vinegar is to add some vegetable oil. Because oil adds fat, the better alternative is to start with less vinegar and add it gradually until you arrive at a flavor you prefer.

Tangy Lemon-Garlic Tomato Dressing

PER SERVING: Calories: 7 | Protein: 0g | Carbohydrates: 1g | Fat: 1g | Saturated Fat: 0g
Cholesterol: 0mg | Sodium: 1mg | Fiber: 1g | PCF Ratio: 14-44-42 | Exchange Approx.: ½ Free

INGREDIENTS | YIELDS ABOUT ¾ CUP; SERVING SIZE: 1 TABLESPOON

1 tablespoon ground flaxseeds
2 cloves garlic
⅛ cup cider vinegar
⅛ teaspoon freshly ground pepper
1 small tomato, chopped
¼ teaspoon celery seed
1 tablespoon lemon juice
¼ cup water

Place all ingredients in blender; blend until smooth.

Friendly Fat and Fiber

In addition to providing fiber, ground flaxseeds are rich sources of omega-3 and -6 essential fatty acids. The oil is low in saturated fat and therefore a heart-healthy choice. Just remember that flaxseed oil must be refrigerated or it will go rancid.

Cashew-Garlic Ranch Dressing

PER SERVING: Calories: 21 | Protein: 1g | Carbohydrates: 2g | Fat: 2g | Saturated Fat: 0g
Cholesterol: 0mg | Sodium: 14mg | Fiber: 0g | PCF Ratio: 10-33-57 | Exchange Approx.: ½ Fat

INGREDIENTS | YIELDS ABOUT ¾ CUP; SERVING SIZE: 1 TABLESPOON

¼ cup raw cashews, or ⅛ cup cashew butter without salt
½ cup water
½ teaspoon stone-ground mustard
1½ tablespoons chili sauce
½ teaspoon horseradish
1 teaspoon Bragg's Liquid Aminos, or tamari sauce
1 clove garlic
1½ teaspoons honey
⅛ teaspoon pepper

1. Process cashews and water in blender or food processor until creamy.

2. Add remaining ingredients; mix well. Refrigerate for 30 minutes.

Lemon-Almond Dressing

PER SERVING: Calories: 25 | Protein: 1g | Carbohydrates: 2g | Fat: 2g | Saturated Fat: 0g
Cholesterol: 0mg | Sodium: 0mg | Fiber: 1g | PCF Ratio: 12-27-61 | Exchange Approx.: ½ Fat

INGREDIENTS | YIELDS ABOUT ⅔ CUP; SERVING SIZE: 1 TABLESPOON

¼ cup raw almonds

1 tablespoon lemon juice

¼ cup water

1½ teaspoons honey

¼ teaspoon lemon pepper

½ slice (1" diameter) peeled ginger

¼ clove garlic

1½ teaspoons chopped fresh chives, or ½ teaspoon dried chives

1½ teaspoons chopped fresh sweet basil, or ½ teaspoon dried basil

Put all ingredients in food processor or blender; process until smooth.

Salad: Undressed

Make a quick salad without dressing by mixing chopped celery, onion, and other vegetables such as cucumbers or zucchini. Add low-salt seasoning or toss vegetables with Bragg's Liquid Aminos or low-sodium soy sauce and serve over salad greens.

Caribbean Kiwi Salsa

PER SERVING: Calories: 79 | Protein: 2g | Carbohydrates: 19g | Fat: 0g | Saturated Fat: 0g | Cholesterol: 0mg
Sodium: 28mg | Fiber: 3g | PCF Ratio: 9-87-5 | Exchange Approx.: 1 Fruit, ½ Vegetable

INGREDIENTS | SERVES 6

1 cup kiwi, peeled and chopped

1 cup pineapple, chopped

1 cup mango, peeled and chopped

⅓ cup red onion, chopped

1 cup red bell pepper, chopped

⅓ cup black beans, cooked

3 tablespoons fresh cilantro, chopped

2 tablespoons lime juice

½ teaspoon chili powder

Dash cayenne

1. Mix all ingredients together in medium bowl.

2. Chill at least 2 hours before serving.

Zesty Black Bean Salsa

PER SERVING, without salt: Calories: 91 | Protein: 4g | Carbohydrates: 13g | Fat: 3g
Saturated Fat: 0g | Cholesterol: 0mg | Sodium: 125mg | Fiber: 4g | PCF Ratio: 15-55-30
Exchange Approx.: ½ Starch, 1 Vegetable, ½ Fat

INGREDIENTS | SERVES 10

1 cup red onion, chopped
¼ cup cilantro, chopped
¼ cup parsley, chopped
3 tablespoons jalapeño, chopped
1½ cups black beans, cooked
4 cups tomato, chopped
3 tablespoons lime juice
2 tablespoons olive oil

1. Place onion, cilantro, parsley, and jalapeño in food processor; chop finely.

2. In medium bowl, combine onion mixture, black beans, and tomatoes.

3. In small bowl, whisk together lime juice and olive oil. Pour over ingredients; mix well.

4. Chill well before serving.

Fresh Peach-Mango Salsa

PER SERVING: Calories: 45 | Protein: 1g | Carbohydrates: 10g | Fat: 1g | Saturated Fat: 0g
Cholesterol: 0mg | Sodium: 104mg | Fiber: 2g | PCF Ratio: 9-82-9 | Exchange Approx.: ½ Fruit

INGREDIENTS | SERVES 6

1 cup mango, peeled and cut into ¼" pieces
1 peach, peeled and cut into ¼" pieces
1 cup red onion, finely chopped
1 cup cucumber, peeled and cut into ¼" pieces
1 tablespoon balsamic vinegar
1 tablespoon lime juice
1 teaspoon chili powder
½ teaspoon cumin
1 tablespoon fresh cilantro, chopped
1 tablespoon parsley, chopped
¼ teaspoon salt

1. Mix all ingredients together in medium bowl.

2. Chill at least 4 hours before serving.

Pineapple-Chili Salsa

PER SERVING: Calories: 29 | Protein: 1g | Carbohydrates: 7g | Fat: 0g | Saturated Fat: 0g
Cholesterol: 0mg | Sodium: 2mg | Fiber: 1g | PCF Ratio: 8-87-5 | Exchange Approx.: ½ Fruit

INGREDIENTS | SERVES 4

½ cup unsweetened diced pineapple

½ cup roughly chopped papaya, peach, or mango

1 small poblano chili pepper

¼ cup chopped red bell pepper

¼ cup chopped yellow bell pepper

1 tablespoon fresh key lime or fresh lime juice

¼ cup chopped red onion

Combine all ingredients in bowl; toss to mix.

Salsa with a Kick

PER SERVING: Calories: 5 | Protein: 0g | Carbohydrates: 1g | Fat: 0g | Saturated Fat: 0g | Cholesterol: 0mg
Sodium: 2mg | Fiber: 0g | PCF Ratio: 14-65-21 | Exchange Approx.: 3 tablespoons = 1 Free Condiment

INGREDIENTS | YIELDS ABOUT 2 CUPS; SERVING SIZE: 1 TABLESPOON

2 teaspoons ground flaxseed

4 medium tomatoes, chopped

1 clove garlic, chopped

½ of small onion

½ tablespoon cider vinegar

¼ teaspoon Tabasco sauce

⅛ teaspoon ground cayenne pepper

1 tablespoon chopped fresh coriander

Place all ingredients in blender or food processor; process briefly, until blended but not smooth.

Avocado-Corn Salsa

PER SERVING: Calories: 133 | Protein: 2g | Carbohydrates: 14g | Fat: 9g | Saturated Fat: 1g | Cholesterol: 0mg
Sodium: 10mg | Fiber: 4g | PCF Ratio: 7-37-56 | Exchange Approx.: ½ Starch/Vegetable, 2 Fats

INGREDIENTS | SERVES 4

1 cup corn kernels, blanched fresh or thawed frozen

1 small banana pepper, seeded and chopped

¼ cup diced red radishes

⅛ cup thinly sliced green onion

1 avocado, diced

1 tablespoon lime juice

½ teaspoon white wine vinegar

1 teaspoon extra-virgin olive oil

¼ teaspoon dried oregano

Dash of ground cumin

Dash of Tabasco sauce

Freshly ground black pepper (optional)

1. Combine corn, banana pepper, radish, and green onion in medium bowl.

2. In another bowl, combine half of diced avocado and lime juice; stir to thoroughly coat.

3. In blender, combine other ½ of avocado, vinegar, oil, oregano, cumin, and Tabasco; process until smooth. Pour over corn mixture; stir.

4. Add avocado mixture. Serve immediately.

Cranberry Orange Relish

PER SERVING: Calories: 62 | Protein: 0g | Carbohydrates: 16g | Fat: 0g | Saturated Fat: 0g
Cholesterol: 0mg | Sodium: 3mg | Fiber: 2g | PCF Ratio: 3-96-1 | Exchange Approx.: 1 Fruit

INGREDIENTS | SERVES 12; SERVING SIZE: ½ CUP

16 ounces fresh cranberries

1½ cups orange sections

2 teaspoons orange zest

¼ cup brown sugar

⅓ cup Splenda Granular

1 teaspoon cinnamon

1. Chop cranberries and orange sections in food processor using pulse setting until coarsely chopped. Transfer to saucepan.

2. Bring cranberry mixture, orange zest, brown sugar, and Splenda to boil over medium heat. Cook 2 minutes.

3. Remove from heat, stir in cinnamon. Chill before serving.

Horseradish Mustard

PER SERVING: Calories: 10 | Protein: 0g | Carbohydrates: 1g | Fat: 1g | Saturated Fat: 0g
Cholesterol: 0mg | Sodium: 68mg | Fiber: 0g | PCF Ratio: 12-25-63 | Exchange Approx.: 1 Free Condiment

INGREDIENTS | YIELDS ¾ CUP; SERVING SIZE: 1 TEASPOON

¼ cup dry mustard

2½ tablespoons prepared horseradish

1 teaspoon sea salt

¼ cup white wine vinegar

1 tablespoon olive oil

Cayenne pepper, to taste (optional)

Combine ingredients in food processor or blender; process until smooth. Pour into decorative jar; store in refrigerator.

Roasted Corn Salsa

PER SERVING: Calories: 104 | Protein: 4g | Carbohydrates: 24g | Fat: 1g | Saturated Fat: 0g | Cholesterol: 0mg
Sodium: 77mg | Fiber: 3g | PCF Ratio: 12-80-8 | Exchange Approx.: 1 Starch, ½ Vegetable

INGREDIENTS | SERVES 6

2 ears corn

1½ cups fresh tomatoes, skinned and chopped

½ cup red onion, chopped

3 tablespoons jalapeño pepper, finely chopped

1 tablespoon rice wine vinegar

¼ cup roasted red pepper, chopped

1½ tablespoons cilantro, chopped

1 teaspoon garlic, finely chopped

1 tablespoon lime juice

½ teaspoon cumin

2 teaspoons red wine vinegar

1. Husk corn and place on grill. Cook for about 10–12 minutes until lightly browned and tender. Set aside to cool.

2. Combine tomatoes, onion, jalapeño, rice wine vinegar, red pepper, cilantro, garlic, lime juice, cumin, and vinegar.

3. When corn has cooled, cut kernels off cobb and add to remaining ingredients.

Pepper and Corn Relish

PER SERVING: Calories: 39 | Protein: 2g | Carbohydrates: 9g | Fat: 1g | Saturated Fat: 0g
Cholesterol: 0mg | Sodium: 7mg | Fiber: 2g | PCF Ratio: 14-78-8 | Exchange Approx.: ½ Starch

INGREDIENTS | SERVES 4; SERVING SIZE: ½ CUP

4 banana or jalapeño peppers
⅓ cup frozen corn, thawed
⅓ cup chopped red onion
⅛ teaspoon ground coriander
2 teaspoons lime juice
Freshly ground black pepper, to taste

Seed and chop peppers; toss in bowl with remaining ingredients. Relish can be served immediately, or chilled and served the next day.

Tip

For a colorful mild relish, use a combination of 2 tablespoons chopped green bell pepper and an equal amount of chopped red pepper in place of the jalapeño peppers.

Plum Sauce

PER SERVING: Calories: 29 | Protein: 0g | Carbohydrates: 8g | Fat: 0g | Saturated Fat: 0g
Cholesterol: 0mg | Sodium: 0mg | Fiber: 0g | PCF Ratio: 0-100-0 | Exchange Approx.: ½ Fruit

INGREDIENTS | YIELDS 1¼ CUPS; SERVING SIZE: 1 TABLESPOON

1 cup plum jam
2 teaspoons grated lemon zest
1 tablespoon lemon juice
1 tablespoon rice wine vinegar
½ teaspoon ground ginger
½ teaspoon crushed anise seeds
¼ teaspoon dry mustard
¼ teaspoon ground cinnamon
⅛ teaspoon ground cloves
⅛ teaspoon hot pepper sauce

1. Heat plum jam in small saucepan over medium heat until melted.

2. Stir in remaining ingredients. Bring the mixture to a boil; lower heat and simmer for 1 minute, stirring constantly. Use cooled sauce as meat seasoning or a dip for eggrolls.

Homemade Worcestershire Sauce

PER SERVING: Calories: 14 | Protein: 0g | Carbohydrates: 4g | Fat: 0g | Saturated Fat: 0g
Cholesterol: 0mg | Sodium: 15mg | Fiber: 0g | PCF Ratio: 3-97-0 | Exchange Approx.: 1 Free Condiment

INGREDIENTS | YIELDS 1 CUP; SERVING SIZE: 1 TABLESPOON

1½ cups cider vinegar
¼ cup plum jam
1 tablespoon blackstrap molasses
1 clove garlic, crushed
⅛ teaspoon chili powder
⅛ teaspoon ground cloves
Pinch of cayenne pepper
¼ cup chopped onion
½ teaspoon ground allspice
⅛ teaspoon dry mustard
1 teaspoon Bragg's Liquid Aminos

Combine all ingredients in large saucepan; stir until mixture boils. Lower heat; simmer uncovered for 1 hour, stirring occasionally. Store in covered jar in refrigerator.

Gingered Peach Sauce

PER SERVING: Calories: 54 | Protein: 1g | Carbohydrates: 5g | Fat: 2g | Saturated Fat: 1g
Cholesterol: 0mg | Sodium: 57mg | Fiber: 1g | PCF Ratio: 5-47-48 | Exchange Approx.: ½ Fat, 1 Fruit

INGREDIENTS | SERVES 4; SERVING SIZE: ½ CUP

2 teaspoons olive oil
1 tablespoon chopped shallot
2 teaspoons grated fresh ginger
⅓ cup dry white wine
1 small peach, peeled and diced
1 tablespoon frozen unsweetened orange juice concentrate
1 teaspoon Bragg's Liquid Aminos
½ teaspoon cornstarch

1. Heat olive oil in nonstick skillet over medium heat; sauté shallot and ginger. Add wine; simmer until reduced by half. Add peach, orange juice concentrate, and Bragg's Liquid Aminos; return to simmer, stirring occasionally.

2. In separate container, mix cornstarch with a tablespoon of sauce; stir to create a slurry, mixing well to remove any lumps. Add slurry to sauce; simmer for 5–7 minutes until mixture thickens. Transfer to blender or food processor; process until smooth.

Fat-Free Roux

PER SERVING, roux only: Calories: 13 | Protein: 0g | Carbohydrates: 2g | Fat: 0g | Saturated Fat: 0g
Cholesterol: 0mg | Sodium: 1mg | Fiber: 0g | PCF Ratio: 1-99-0 | Exchange Approx.: 1 Free

INGREDIENTS | YIELDS ENOUGH TO THICKEN 1 CUP OF LIQUID; SERVING SIZE: ¼ CUP

1 tablespoon cornstarch
2 tablespoons wine
(Make this roux with red wine for a defatted beef broth gravy. Use white wine for chicken or seafood gravy or sauce.)

1. Whisk ingredients together until well blended, making sure there are no lumps.

2. To use as thickener for 1 cup of broth, heat broth until it reaches a boil. Slowly whisk cornstarch-wine mixture into broth; return to a boil. Reduce heat; simmer, stirring constantly, until mixture thickens enough to coat back of spoon. (A gravy or sauce made in this manner will thicken more as it cools. It's important to bring a cornstarch slurry to a boil; this helps it thicken and removes the starchy taste.)

Mock Béchamel Sauce

PER SERVING: Calories: 53 | Protein: 4g | Carbohydrates: 4g | Fat: 2g | Saturated Fat: 1g
Cholesterol: 51mg | Sodium: 58mg | Fiber: 0g | PCF Ratio: 32-32-36 | Exchange Approx.: ½ Fat, ½ Skim Milk

INGREDIENTS | YIELDS 1 CUP; SERVING SIZE: ¼ CUP

1 egg
1 cup Mock Cream (page 183)
1 teaspoon unsalted butter

1. In quart-size or larger microwave-safe bowl, whisk egg into Mock Cream until well blended. Microwave on high for 1 minute; whisk mixture again. Microwave on high for 30 seconds; whisk again. Microwave on high for another 30 seconds; whisk again. (Strain mixture if there appears to be any cooked egg solids; this seldom occurs if mixture is whisked at intervals specified.)

2. Allow the mixture to cool slightly; whisk in butter.

Piccalilli

PER SERVING, without salt: Calories: 13 | Protein: 0g | Carbohydrates: 3g | Fat: 0g
Saturated Fat: 0g | Cholesterol: 0mg | Sodium: 1mg | Fiber: 0g | PCF Ratio: 4-94-1
Exchange Approx. (per ⅛ cup serving): ½ Misc. Carbohydrate

**INGREDIENTS | YIELDS 2 QUARTS;
SERVING SIZE: 2
TABLESPOONS**

1 cup chopped green tomatoes

1½ cups chopped cabbage

1 cup white onions

1 cup chopped cauliflower

1 cup chopped cucumber

½ cup chopped red pepper

½ cup chopped green pepper

¼ cup pickling salt

1½ cups apple cider or white vinegar

¾ cup sugar

½ teaspoon turmeric

1 teaspoon ginger

1½ teaspoons dried mustard

1½ teaspoons mustard seed

1 teaspoon celery seed

Sachet of pickling spices

Pickled whole onions, to taste (optional)

1. Dice vegetables and layer in bowl with pickling salt. Store in refrigerator overnight to remove moisture from vegetables.

2. Drain and rinse vegetables. (Rinsing will remove much of the salt; however, if sodium is a concern, you can omit it altogether.)

3. To make marinade, combine vinegar, sugar, turmeric, ginger, dried mustard, mustard seed, celery seed, and pickling spice sachet in large, noncorrosive stockpot. Bring ingredients to boil; boil for 2 minutes. Add vegetables; boil for an additional 10 minutes.

4. Remove pickling spice sachet and add pickled onions, if you are using them; boil for another 2 minutes.

5. Remove from heat and allow to cool. Pack vegetables in jars, then fill with pickling liquid until vegetables are covered. Store covered glass jars in refrigerator. Serve chilled as a relish or on deli sandwiches.

Comparative Analysis

Omitting both sugar and pickling salt makes this recipe even better for you, with ⅓ the calories, less than ½ the carbohydrates, a PCF Ratio of 12-84-4, and an Exchange Approximation of ½ Free Vegetable.

Cranberry-Raisin Chutney

PER SERVING, without salt: Calories: 14 | Protein: 0g | Carbohydrates: 3g | Fat: 0g | Saturated Fat: 0g
Cholesterol: 0mg | Sodium: 1mg | Fiber: 0g | PCF Ratio: 4-93-3 | Exchange Approx.: 1 Free Condiment

INGREDIENTS | YIELDS ABOUT 3 CUPS; SERVING SIZE: 1 TABLESPOON

1 cup diced onions

1 cup diced peeled apples

1 cup diced bananas

1 cup diced peaches

¼ cup raisins

¼ cup dry white wine

¼ cup American Spoon Foods Dried Cranberries

¼ cup apple cider vinegar

1 teaspoon brown sugar

Sea salt and freshly ground black pepper, to taste (optional)

In large saucepan, combine all ingredients. Cook over low heat for about 1 hour, stirring occasionally. Cool completely. Can be kept for a week in refrigerator or in freezer for 3 months, or canned using same sterilizing method you'd use to can mincemeat.

Tip

This chutney is also good if you substitute other dried fruit for the raisins or cranberries, such as using the dried Fancy Fruit Mix from Nutty Guys (*www.nuttyguys.com*).

Roasted Red Pepper and Plum Sauce

PER SERVING: Calories: 38 | Protein: 0g | Carbohydrates: 10g | Fat: 1g | Saturated Fat: 0g | Cholesterol: 0mg
Sodium: 76mg | Fiber: 1g | PCF Ratio: 3-95-2 | Exchange Approx.: ½ Misc. Carbohydrate

INGREDIENTS | YIELDS 2 CUPS; SERVING SIZE: 1 TABLESPOON

1 large roasted red pepper, pulp only (see sidebar)

½ pound apricots, quartered and pitted

¾ pound plums, quartered and pitted

1⅓ cups apple cider vinegar

⅔ cup water

⅓ cup white sugar

½ cup brown sugar

2 tablespoons corn syrup

2 tablespoons fresh grated ginger

1 teaspoon salt

1 tablespoon toasted mustard seeds

4 scallions, chopped (white part only)

1 teaspoon minced garlic

½ teaspoon ground cinnamon

1. Place all ingredients together in large pot; bring to a boil. Reduce heat; simmer, covered, for 30 minutes.

2. Uncover and simmer for another hour.

3. Place in blender or food processor; process to desired consistency. Can be stored in refrigerator for 4–6 weeks.

Roasting Red Peppers

The traditional method of roasting a red pepper is to use a long-handled fork to hold the pepper over the open flame of a gas burner until it's charred. Of course, there are a variety of other methods as well. You can place the pepper on a rack set over an electric burner and turn it occasionally, until the skin is blackened. This should take about 4 to 6 minutes. You can also put the pepper over direct heat on a preheated grill. Use tongs to turn the pepper occasionally. Another method is to broil the pepper on a broiler rack about 2 inches from the heat, turning the pepper every five minutes. Total broiling time will be about 15 to 20 minutes, or until the skins are blistered and charred. The key to peeling the peppers is letting them sit in their steam in a closed container until they are cool. Once the peppers are cool, the skin will rub or peel off easily.

Pesto Sauce

PER SERVING: Calories: 37 | Protein: 1g | Carbohydrates: 1g | Fat: 4g | Saturated Fat: 1g
Cholesterol: 1mg | Sodium: 14mg | Fiber: 0g | PCF Ratio: 10-6-85 | Exchange Approx.: 1 Fat

**INGREDIENTS | YIELDS ABOUT 3 CUPS;
SERVING SIZE: 1
TABLESPOON**

¾ cup pine nuts
4 cups tightly packed basil leaves
½ cup freshly grated Parmesan cheese
3 large garlic cloves, minced
¼ teaspoon salt
1 teaspoon freshly ground black pepper
½ cup extra-virgin olive oil

1. Preheat oven to 350°F. Spread pine nuts on baking sheet. Bake for about 5 minutes; stir. Continue to bake for 10 minutes until nuts are golden brown and highly aromatic, stirring occasionally. Let nuts cool completely; chop finely.

2. Fill medium-sized heavy saucepan halfway with water. Place over medium heat; bring to a boil. Next to pot, place large bowl filled with water and ice. Using tongs, dip a few basil leaves into boiling water. Blanch for 3 seconds; quickly remove from boiling water and place in ice water. Repeat process until all basil has been blanched, adding ice to water as needed. Drain basil in colander and pat dry with a towel.

3. In blender or food processor, combine basil, pine nuts, cheese, garlic, salt, pepper, and all but 1 tablespoon olive oil; process until smooth and uniform. Pour into airtight container and add remaining olive oil to top to act as protective barrier. Pesto can be stored in refrigerator for up to 5 days.

4. To freeze pesto, place it in a tightly sealed container. To freeze small amounts of pesto, pour into ice cube trays and freeze until solid. Once frozen, you can remove the pesto cubes and place them in sealed freezer bags.

Mock White Sauce

PER RECIPE: Calories: 61 | Protein: 2g | Carbohydrates: 6g | Fat: 3g | Saturated Fat: 2g
Cholesterol: 9mg | Sodium: 190mg | Fiber: 0g | PCF Ratio: 20-36-44 | Exchange Approx.: ½ Fat, ½ Skim Milk

**INGREDIENTS | YIELDS ABOUT 1 CUP;
SERVING SIZE: ½ CUP**

1 tablespoon unsalted butter
1 tablespoon flour
¼ teaspoon sea salt
Pinch of white pepper
1 cup Mock Cream (page 183)

1. In medium-sized heavy nonstick saucepan, melt butter over very low heat. Butter should gently melt; you do not want it to bubble and turn brown. While butter is melting, mix together flour, salt, and white pepper in small bowl.

2. Once butter is melted, add flour mixture; stir constantly. (A heat-safe flat-bottom spoon safe for nonstick pans works well for this.) Once mixture thickens and starts to bubble, about 2 minutes, slowly pour in some Mock Cream; stir until blended with roux. Add a little more Mock Cream; stir until blended. Add remaining Mock Cream; continue cooking, stirring constantly to make sure sauce doesn't stick to bottom of pan. Once sauce begins to steam and appears it's just about to boil, reduce heat and simmer until sauce thickens, or about 3 minutes.

Madeira Sauce

PER SERVING: Calories: 56 | Protein: 0g | Carbohydrates: 2g | Fat: 4g | Saturated Fat: 2g
Cholesterol: 5mg | Sodium: 3mg | Fiber: 0g | PCF Ratio: 2-14-84 | Exchange Approx.: 1 Fat, ½ Vegetable

INGREDIENTS | SERVES 4; SERVING SIZE: ¼ CUP

2 teaspoons olive oil

1 clove garlic, crushed

1 tablespoon chopped shallot

1 teaspoon unsalted tomato paste

⅓ cup Madeira

¼ cup shellfish, vegetable, or chicken broth

1 tablespoon lemon juice

2 teaspoons Mock Cream (page 183)

2 teaspoons unsalted butter

Salt and freshly ground black pepper (optional)

1. Heat olive oil in nonstick saucepan over medium heat. Add garlic and shallot; sauté for 3 minutes until translucent.

2. Add tomato paste; sauté 30 seconds, stirring as needed.

3. Add Madeira, broth, lemon juice, and Mock Cream; simmer for 5 minutes until mixture is reduced by half. Whisk in butter to form an emulsion. (Optional: Strain sauce and season with salt and pepper.)

Tip

Keep the sauce warm until needed, being careful not to let it boil or become too cold after the butter has been added.

Mock Cauliflower Sauce

PER SERVING: Calories: 27 | Protein: 2g | Carbohydrates: 5g | Fat: 1g | Saturated Fat: 0g | Cholesterol: 0mg
Sodium: 16mg | Fiber: 2g | PCF Ratio: 24-66-10 | Exchange Approx.: 1 Vegetable

INGREDIENTS | SERVES 4; SERVING SIZE: ½ CUP

2 cups cauliflower

¼ cup diced Spanish onion

1 clove roasted garlic (see Dry-Roasted Garlic on page 26), or ½ clove crushed garlic

1 tablespoon dry white wine

Freshly ground white pepper, to taste

⅛ cup (2 tablespoons) Mock Cream (page 183)

1. Add cauliflower, onion, garlic, and white wine to microwave-safe bowl; cover and microwave on high for 5 minutes, or until cauliflower is tender and onions are transparent. (Microwave on high for additional 1-minute intervals, if necessary.)

2. Pour vegetable-wine mixture into blender or food processor, being careful not to burn yourself on steam. Season with white pepper and add Mock Cream; process until smooth.

Tip

If you use frozen cauliflower to make Mock Cauliflower Sauce, be sure to thaw and drain it first. Otherwise, there will be too much moisture and the resulting sauce will be too thin.

CHAPTER 13

Yeast Breads, Quick Breads, and Muffins

Hawaiian-Style Bread

PER SERVING: Calories: 89 | Protein: 2g | Carbohydrates: 17g | Fat: 1g | Saturated Fat: 1g
Cholesterol: 11mg | Sodium: 103mg | Fiber: 1g | PCF Ratio: 11-75-14 | Exchange Approx.: 1 Starch

INGREDIENTS | YIELDS 1 LARGE LOAF, 24 SLICES; SERVING SIZE: 1 SLICE

1 egg

½ cup pineapple juice, or ⅛ cup frozen pineapple juice concentrate and ⅜ cup water

¾ cup water

2 tablespoons butter

1 teaspoon vanilla

½ teaspoon dried ginger

1 teaspoon salt

1½ cups unbleached bread flour

2⅛ cups unbleached all-purpose flour

¼ cup sugar

2 tablespoons nonfat milk powder

1 package (2½ teaspoons) active dry yeast

Unless instructions for bread machine differ, add ingredients in order listed here. Use light-crust setting.

Bread Machine White Bread

PER SERVING: Calories: 90 | Protein: 3g | Carbohydrates: 17g | Fat: 1g | Saturated Fat: 0g
Cholesterol: 1mg | Sodium: 106mg | Fiber: 1g | PCF Ratio: 13-79-8 | Exchange Approx.: 1 Starch

INGREDIENTS | YIELDS 1 LARGE LOAF; SERVING SIZE: 1 SLICE

1¼ cups skim milk

2 tablespoons nonfat milk powder

1 tablespoon olive or canola oil

1 teaspoon sea salt

1 tablespoon granulated sugar

4 cups unbleached all-purpose or bread flour

1 package (2½ teaspoons) active dry yeast

Add ingredients to bread machine in order recommended by manufacturer, being careful yeast doesn't come in contact with salt.

Honey Oat Bran Bread

PER SERVING: Calories: 86 | Protein: 3g | Carbohydrates: 16g | Fat: 1g | Saturated Fat: 0g
Cholesterol: 8mg | Sodium: 109mg | Fiber: 1g | PCF Ratio: 15-72-13 | Exchange Approx.: 1 Starch

INGREDIENTS | YIELDS 1 LARGE LOAF;
SERVING SIZE: 1 SLICE

1¼ cups skim milk

2 tablespoons nonfat buttermilk powder

1 tablespoon olive or canola oil

1 medium egg

1 cup oat bran

1 teaspoon sea salt

½ cup whole-wheat flour

2½ cups unbleached all-purpose or bread flour

1 tablespoon honey

1 package (2½ teaspoons) active dry yeast

Use light-crust setting on your bread machine; add ingredients in order recommended by manufacturer. Be careful yeast doesn't come in contact with salt.

7-Grain Bread

PER SERVING: Calories: 82 | Protein: 3g | Carbohydrates: 15g | Fat: 1g | Saturated Fat: 0g
Cholesterol: 8mg | Sodium: 108mg | Fiber: 1g | PCF Ratio: 14-73-12 | Exchange Approx.: 1 Starch

INGREDIENTS | YIELD: 1 LARGE LOAF;
SERVING SIZE: 1 SLICE

1¼ cups skim milk

2 tablespoons nonfat milk powder

1 tablespoon olive or canola oil

¾ cup dry 7-grain cereal

½ cup oat bran

1 teaspoon sea salt

2¼ cups unbleached all-purpose or bread flour

½ cup whole-wheat flour

1 tablespoon honey

1 package (2½ teaspoons) dry yeast

Add ingredients to bread machine in order recommended by manufacturer, being careful that yeast doesn't come in contact with salt. Bake on whole-wheat bread setting.

Lactose-Free Bread

When cooking for someone who is lactose intolerant, substitute equal amounts of water or soy milk for any milk called for in bread recipes.

Cheddar Cornbread

PER SERVING: Calories: 102 | Protein: 3g | Carbohydrates: 16g | Fat: 3g | Saturated Fat: 2g
Cholesterol: 8mg | Sodium: 172mg | Fiber: 1g | PCF Ratio: 13-63-24 | Exchange Approx.: 1 Starch, ½ Fat

**INGREDIENTS | YIELDS 1 LARGE LOAF;
SERVING SIZE: 1 SLICE**

1¼ cups water

1 tablespoon honey

3 tablespoons butter

¼ cup nonfat milk powder

1 package (2½ teaspoons) active dry yeast

2½ cups unbleached all-purpose or bread flour

1 cup yellow cornmeal

1½ teaspoons sea salt

⅔ cup grated Cheddar cheese

1. Use light-crust setting. Add all ingredients except cheese in order suggested by bread machine manual. Process on basic bread cycle according to manufacturer's directions.

2. At beeper (or end of first kneading), add cheese.

Cottage Cheese Bread

PER SERVING: Calories: 76 | Protein: 3g | Carbohydrates: 13g | Fat: 1g | Saturated Fat: 1g
Cholesterol: 11mg | Sodium: 114mg | Fiber: 1g | PCF Ratio: 16-68-16 | Exchange Approx.: 1 Starch

**INGREDIENTS | YIELDS 1 LARGE LOAF;
SERVING SIZE: 1 SLICE**

¼ cup water

1 cup nonfat cottage cheese

2 tablespoons butter

1 egg

1 tablespoon sugar

¼ teaspoon baking soda

1 teaspoon salt

3 cups unbleached all-purpose or bread flour

1 package (2½ teaspoons) active dry yeast

Add ingredients in order recommended by manufacturer, being careful yeast doesn't come in contact with salt. Check bread machine at "beep" to make sure dough is pulling away from sides of pan and forming a ball. Add water or flour, if needed. (Note: You do not want dough to be overly dry.) Bake at white bread setting, light crust.

Why Breads Need Salt

Salt is only used in bread to enhance the flavor. If salt comes directly in contact with yeast before yeast has had a chance to begin to work, it can hinder the action of the yeast. Keep that in mind when adding ingredients to your bread machine.

Basic White Bread

PER SERVING: Calories: 77 | Protein: 2g | Carbohydrates: 15g | Fat: 1g | Saturated Fat: 0g
Cholesterol: 0mg | Sodium: 175mg | Fiber: 1g | PCF Ratio: 11-79-10 | Exchange Approx.: 1 Starch

INGREDIENTS | **YIELDS 2 LARGE LOAVES; SERVING SIZE: 1 SLICE**

5½–6 cups flour

1 package (2½ teaspoons) active dry yeast

¼ cup warm water

2 tablespoons sugar

1¾ cups warm water

2 tablespoons shortening

1 tablespoon sea salt

1. Place ⅓ of flour in large bowl and set aside. Mix yeast with ¼ cup warm water in another bowl, stirring well. Add sugar and water to yeast. Add mixture to flour; stir well. Set aside 5 minutes to allow yeast to proof.

2. Stir; cut in shortening using a pastry blender or your hands. Stir in salt and as much of remaining flour as possible. Dough has enough flour when it's still somewhat sticky to the touch, yet pulls away from side of bowl as it's stirred. Turn dough onto lightly floured work surface. Knead for 8–10 minutes, until smooth and elastic, adding flour as necessary. Dough will take on an almost glossy appearance once it's been kneaded sufficiently.

3. Transfer dough to bowl treated with nonstick spray. Cover with damp cloth; place in warm, draft-free area. Allow to rise until double in volume, about 1–1½ hours.

4. Punch dough down and let rise a second time, until almost doubled in bulk.

5. Treat two 9" × 5" bread pans with nonstick spray. Punch dough down again; divide into 2 loaves. Shape loaves; place in bread pans. Cover and let rise until almost doubled.

6. Preheat oven to 350°F. Bake 20–30 minutes, or until golden brown. Remove from pans and allow to cool on rack.

Fiber-Enriched Cheddar Bread

PER SERVING: Calories: 141 | Protein: 6g | Carbohydrates: 25g | Fat: 1g | Saturated Fat: 0g
Cholesterol: 2mg | Sodium: 546mg | Fiber: 1g | PCF Ratio: 19-73-8 | Exchange Approx.: 1½ Starches

INGREDIENTS | YIELDS 1 LOAF (12 SLICES); SERVING SIZE: 1 SLICE

1½ cups warm water

1 package (2½ teaspoons) active dry yeast

2½ teaspoons salt

½ cup wheat bran

3 cups bread flour

⅔ cups reduced-fat Cheddar cheese, grated

1 tablespoon Parmesan cheese

Cornmeal for cookie sheet

1. Combine water, yeast, and salt in mixer bowl or food processor. Add remaining ingredients; mix well using dough hook or dough attachment until very soft dough is formed.

2. Transfer dough to large, loosely covered bowl; allow to rise at room temperature for 2 hours. Dough can be used after rising, but is much easier to handle after it has been refrigerated several hours or overnight.

3. When ready to bake, sprinkle a light dusting of flour on top of dough. With floured hands, remove dough from bowl; shape into round loaf.

4. Place dough on cookie sheet or pizza peel liberally covered with cornmeal. Allow dough to rise at room temperature for 45 minutes.

5. Preheat oven to 450°F with baking or pizza stone placed in center rack of oven. Before transferring dough to hot stone, slash dough across top using floured sharp knife. Slide dough onto hot baking stone; place shallow pan of hot water on lower rack of oven to create steam underneath bread.

6. Bake for 40 minutes, or until bread is deeply browned and has a hardened crust. Remove to a cooling rack; allow to cool before slicing.

Golden Raisin Bread

PER SERVING: Calories: 163 | Protein: 6g | Carbohydrates: 34g | Fat: 1g | Saturated Fat: 0g
Cholesterol: 0mg | Sodium: 497mg | Fiber: 3g | PCF Ratio: 13-82-5 | Exchange Approx.: 1½ Starches; ½ Fruit

INGREDIENTS | YIELDS 1 LOAF (12 SLICES); SERVING SIZE: 1 SLICE

1½ cups warm water

2½ teaspoons active dry yeast

2½ teaspoons salt

⅓ cup wheat germ

1 cup whole-wheat flour

2 cups bread flour

2 tablespoons honey

1 teaspoon cinnamon

½ cup golden raisins

1 tablespoon egg white

½ tablespoon water

Tools of the Trade

Nonstick pans with a dark surface absorb too much heat, which causes breads to burn. Chicago Metallic makes muffin, mini-muffin, and other bread pans with lighter-colored Silverstone nonstick coating that are much better suited for baking.

1. Combine water, yeast, and salt in mixer bowl or food processor. Using dough hook or dough attachment for food processor, add in remaining ingredients except egg white and water; mix well until very soft dough is formed.

2. Transfer dough to loosely covered large bowl; allow to rise at room temperature for 2 hours. Dough can be used after rising; however, it is much easier to handle after it has been refrigerated several hours or overnight.

3. When ready to bake, lightly grease 9" × 4" × 3" loaf pan. Scoop dough out of bowl with wet hands (this makes it easier to handle); shape into elongated loaf and place in loaf pan. Allow dough to rise for 1 hour.

4. Preheat oven to 375°F. Brush loaf with egg wash of 1 tablespoon of egg white and ½ tablespoon water.

5. Bake on middle rack of preheated oven. Place shallow pan of hot water on the lower rack to create steam under bread.

6. Bake for 45–50 minutes, until bread is golden brown. Cool in pan for 10 minutes, then remove to wire rack. Allow bread to cool completely before slicing.

Whole-Wheat Bread

PER SERVING: Calories: 86 | Protein: 2g | Carbohydrates: 17g | Fat: 1g | Saturated Fat: 0g
Cholesterol: 0mg | Sodium: 118mg | Fiber: 1g | PCF Ratio: 10-77-13 | Exchange Approx.: 1 Starch

INGREDIENTS | YIELDS 2 LOAVES; SERVING SIZE: 1 SLICE

1 package (2½ teaspoons) active dry yeast

2 cups warm water

3 cups unbleached all-purpose or bread flour

2 tablespoons sugar

½ cup hot water

2 teaspoons salt

½ cup brown sugar

3 tablespoons shortening

3 cups whole-wheat flour

History Lesson

The sponge process of making bread was more popular years ago, when foodstuffs were less processed and the quality of yeast was less reliable. The yeast works in a batter and the dough rises only once. The sponge process produces a loaf that is lighter but coarser grained.

1. Add yeast to 2 cups warm water. Stir in all-purpose flour and sugar; beat until smooth, either by hand or with mixer. Set in warm place to proof until it becomes foamy and bubbly, up to 1 hour.

2. Combine ½ cup hot water, salt, brown sugar, and shortening; stir. Allow to cool to lukewarm. (Stirring sugar until it's dissolved should be sufficient to cool water; test to be sure, as adding liquid that's too warm can kill yeast.) Add to bubbly flour mixture. Stir in whole-wheat flour; beat until smooth, but do not knead.

3. Divide dough into 2 lightly greased pans. Cover; set in warm place until doubled in size. Preheat oven to 350°F; bake for 50 minutes.

Multigrain Cornbread

PER SERVING: Calories: 124 | Protein: 4g | Carbohydrates: 20g | Fat: 3g | Saturated Fat: 1g
Cholesterol: 16mg | Sodium: 220mg | Fiber: 2g | PCF Ratio: 12-65-23 | Exchange Approx.: 1 Starch, ½ Fat

INGREDIENTS | SERVES 16; SERVING SIZE: 1 SLICE

Nonstick cooking spray
1 egg
2 tablespoons egg whites
3 tablespoons butter, melted
1½ cups low fat buttermilk
1 teaspoon vanilla
1¾ cups cornmeal
¾ cup whole-wheat pastry flour
1 tablespoon ground flaxseed
3 tablespoons Splenda granular
1 tablespoon sugar
4 teaspoons baking powder
½ teaspoon baking soda
Pinch salt

1. Preheat oven to 375°F. Spray 8" × 8" square baking pan with nonstick cooking spray.

2. In medium bowl, whisk together egg, egg whites, butter, buttermilk, and vanilla. Set aside.

3. In larger bowl, combine cornmeal, flour, flaxseed, Splenda, sugar, baking powder, baking soda, and salt; mix well.

4. Make well in center of dry ingredients; pour in buttermilk mixture. Mix gently with spoon until all dry ingredients are moistened; do not over mix.

5. Spoon batter into prepared pan. Bake for 25–30 minutes, or until center springs back when lightly touched. Cool on wire rack before slicing into pieces.

Don't Have Buttermilk?

When baking, soured milk is a good substitution for buttermilk. To replace 1 cup of buttermilk in a recipe, stir 1 tablespoon of white vinegar or fresh lemon juice into 1 cup of milk. Let the milk stand for 5 minutes, or until milk thickens.

Fiber-Enriched Banana Bread

PER SERVING: Calories: 65 | Protein: 5g | Carbohydrates: 29g | Fat: 4g | Saturated Fat: 1g
Cholesterol: 22mg | Sodium: 348mg | Fiber: 4g | PCF Ratio: 12-67-21 | Exchange Approx.: 1 Starch, ½ Fruit, 1 Fat

INGREDIENTS | YIELDS 1 LARGE LOAF, 12 SLICES; SERVING SIZE: 1 SLICE

Nonstick cooking spray
½ cup buttermilk
¼ cup wheat bran
1 cup mashed ripe banana
1 egg
¼ cup egg whites
2 tablespoons canola oil
1 teaspoon vanilla
2 tablespoons honey
1¼ cups whole-wheat pastry flour
½ cup all-purpose flour
⅓ cup Splenda granular
1 teaspoon baking soda
1½ teaspoons baking powder
½ teaspoon salt

1. Preheat oven to 375°F. Spray 9" × 4" × 3" loaf pan with nonstick cooking spray.

2. Place buttermilk and wheat bran in medium bowl; allow wheat bran to soak 10 minutes. Stir in banana, egg, egg whites, oil, vanilla, and honey.

3. In larger bowl, sift together flours, Splenda, baking soda, baking powder, and salt; add dry ingredients to banana mixture. Using a large spoon, stir just until dry ingredients are moistened; do not over mix.

4. Spoon batter into prepared loaf pan. Bake for 45 minutes, or until top is lightly browned and inserted toothpick comes out clean. Cool in pan for 10 minutes before removing to wire rack.

Whole-Wheat Zucchini Bread

PER SERVING: Calories: 178 | Protein: 4g | Carbohydrates: 29g | Fat: 6g | Saturated Fat: 1g
Cholesterol: 25mg | Sodium: 243mg | Fiber: 3g | PCF Ratio: 9-63-28 | Exchange Approx.: 1½ Starches, 1 Fat

INGREDIENTS	YIELDS 4 MINI LOAVES, 20 SLICES (5 SLICES PER MINI LOAF); SERVING SIZE: 1 SLICE

Cooking spray

2 eggs

2 tablespoons egg whites

½ cup honey

2 cups zucchini, shredded

⅔ cup unsweetened applesauce

⅓ cup canola oil

2 teaspoons vanilla

2 cups whole-wheat pastry flour

1 cup all-purpose flour

¼ cup Splenda granular

1 teaspoon salt

2 teaspoons baking powder

1 teaspoon baking soda

2 teaspoons cinnamon

½ teaspoons nutmeg

⅓ cup sunflower seeds, toasted

1. Preheat oven to 350°F. Spray 4 aluminum mini loaf pans with cooking spray.

2. In large mixing bowl, beat egg and egg whites until foamy. Mix in honey, zucchini, applesauce, canola oil, and vanilla.

3. In separate mixing bowl, sift together whole-wheat flour, all-purpose flour, Splenda, salt, baking powder, baking soda, cinnamon, and nutmeg.

4. Gradually add dry ingredients to zucchini mixture; mix until all ingredients are combined, but do not over mix. Stir in sunflower seeds.

5. Divide batter evenly into prepared mini loaf pans. Bake for 35–40 minutes, or until tops are browned and inserted toothpick comes out clean.

6. Remove pans to wire rack and cool for 10 minutes before removing from pans. Cool completely before slicing.

Variations

For a variation on this recipe, ⅓ cup dried cranberries, currants, raisins, or chopped nuts can be added in place of the sunflower seeds.

Applesauce Buckwheat Muffins

PER MUFFIN, with crisp topping: Calories: 182 | Protein: 5g | Carbohydrates: 27g | Fat: 7g | Saturated Fat: 1g
Cholesterol: 24mg | Sodium: 302mg | Fiber: 3g | PCF Ratio: 11-56-34 | Exchange Approx.: 1 Starch, ½ Fruit, 1 Fat

INGREDIENTS | YIELDS 12 MUFFINS; SERVING SIZE: 1 MUFFIN

1 cup buttermilk
½ cup applesauce, unsweetened
¼ cup canola oil
1 egg
2 tablespoons egg whites
2 tablespoons maple syrup
1 teaspoon vanilla
1¼ cups whole-wheat pastry flour
¾ cup light buckwheat flour
¼ cup Splenda granular
1½ teaspoons baking powder
1½ teaspoons baking soda
¼ teaspoon salt
2 teaspoons cinnamon
¼ teaspoon allspice

Crisp Topping (optional):
1 tablespoon Splenda Brown Sugar Blend
¼ teaspoon cinnamon
¼ cup oats
2 teaspoons ground flaxseed
1 tablespoon whole-wheat pastry flour
1 tablespoon butter, melted

1. Preheat oven to 375°F. Prepare muffin pan with nonstick cooking spray.

2. In medium bowl, whisk together buttermilk, applesauce, oil, egg, egg whites, maple syrup, and vanilla. In separate bowl, sift together whole-wheat flour, buckwheat flour, Splenda, baking powder, baking soda, salt, and spices. Gradually add dry ingredients to liquid mixture; mix just enough to combine ingredients. Do not over mix. Spoon batter evenly into prepared muffin pan.

3. In small bowl, mix together all ingredients for crisp topping. Sprinkle evenly on top of each muffin.

4. Bake for 20–25 minutes, or until center of muffin springs back when lightly touched. Cool in muffin tin for 5 minutes before removing to wire rack.

Pear Walnut Muffins

PER MUFFIN, with crisp topping: Calories: 195 | Protein: 5g | Carbohydrates: 27g | Fat: 8g | Saturated Fat: 1g
Cholesterol: 24mg | Sodium: 289mg | Fiber: 3g | PCF Ratio: 11-54-35 | Exchange Approx.: 1 Starch, ½ Fruit, 1 Fat

INGREDIENTS | 12 MUFFINS; SERVING SIZE: 1 MUFFIN

1 cup buttermilk

3 tablespoons canola oil

1 egg

2 tablespoons egg whites

⅔ cup pears, peeled and chopped

2 tablespoons honey

1¼ cups whole-wheat pastry flour

¾ cup all-purpose flour

3 tablespoons Splenda granular

1½ teaspoons baking powder

1½ teaspoons baking soda

¼ teaspoon salt

1 teaspoon cinnamon

¼ teaspoon ginger

⅓ cup walnuts, chopped

Crisp Topping (optional):

1 tablespoon Splenda Brown Sugar Blend

Pinch ginger

¼ cup oats

2 teaspoons ground flaxseed

1 tablespoon whole-wheat pastry flour

1 tablespoon butter, melted

1. Preheat oven to 375°F. Prepare muffin pan with nonstick cooking spray.

2. In medium bowl, whisk together buttermilk, oil, egg, egg whites, pears, and honey.

3. In separate bowl, sift together whole-wheat flour, all-purpose flour, Splenda, baking powder, baking soda, salt, spices, and walnuts. Gradually add dry ingredients to liquid mixture; stir just enough to combine ingredients. Do not over mix. Spoon batter evenly into prepared muffin pan.

4. In small bowl, mix together all ingredients for crisp topping. Sprinkle evenly on top of each muffin.

5. Bake for 20–25 minutes, or until center of muffin springs back when lightly touched. Cool in muffin tin for 5 minutes before removing to wire rack.

Whole-Wheat Pastry Flour

Whole-wheat pastry flour is a finer grind of soft white wheat. When used in quick bread and muffin recipes, it delivers more nutrition and fiber than white flour and yields a lighter texture than whole-wheat flour.

Milk Biscuits

PER SERVING: Calories: 98 | Protein: 2g | Carbohydrates: 13g | Fat: 4g | Saturated Fat: 3g
Cholesterol: 11mg | Sodium: 205mg | Fiber: 0g | PCF Ratio: 9-53-38 | Exchange Approx.: 1 Starch; ½ Fat

INGREDIENTS | YIELDS 24 BISCUITS; SERVING SIZE: 1 BISCUIT

3 cups unbleached all-purpose flour
1 teaspoon salt
1½ teaspoons baking soda
1 tablespoon cream of tartar
1 teaspoon baking powder
½ cup butter
1⅓ cups milk

Healthy Substitutions

Despite the downside of all the butter, the upside is these biscuits are so rich you won't even notice they don't contain sugar. Consult your dietitian if you are on a diet to control cholesterol. You can substitute ¼ cup nonfat yogurt for half of the butter in this recipe.

1. Preheat oven to 400°F. For quick mixing, use food processor. Just add all ingredients at once; pulse until just blended. Be careful not to overprocess, as rolls won't be as light.

2. To mix by hand, sift together dry ingredients. Cut in butter using pastry blender or fork until mixture resembles coarse crumbs. Add milk; stir until mixture pulls away from sides of bowl.

3. Use 1 heaping tablespoon for each biscuit, dropping dough onto greased baking sheets. (You can also try pan liners, such as parchment.) Bake until golden brown, about 20–30 minutes.

Angelic Buttermilk Batter Biscuits

PER SERVING: Calories: 74 | Protein: 2g | Carbohydrates: 12g | Fat: 2g | Saturated Fat: 1g
Cholesterol: 6mg | Sodium: 55mg | Fiber: 1g | PCF Ratio: 11-64-26 | Exchange Approx.: 1 Starch

INGREDIENTS | YIELDS 24 BISCUITS; SERVING SIZE: 1 BISCUIT

3 tablespoons nonfat buttermilk powder

2 tablespoons granulated sugar

¾ cup warm water

1 tablespoon active dry yeast

2½ cups unbleached all-purpose flour

½ teaspoon sea salt

½ teaspoon baking powder

¼ cup unsalted butter

¼ cup nonfat plain yogurt

Why Breads Need Sugar

Bread recipes need sugar or sweetener, like honey, to "feed" the yeast. This helps the yeast work, which in turn helps the bread rise.

1. Put buttermilk powder, sugar, and warm water in food processor; process until mixed. Sprinkle yeast over top; pulse once or twice to mix. Allow mixture to sit at room temperature for about 5 minutes, or until yeast begins to bubble. Add all remaining ingredients to food processor; pulse until mixed, being careful not to overprocess dough.

2. Preheat oven to 400°F; drop 1 heaping teaspoon per biscuit onto baking sheet treated with nonstick spray. Set tray in warm place; allow biscuits to rise for about 15 minutes.

3. Bake biscuits for 12–15 minutes.

Orange Date Bread

PER SERVING: Calories: 79 | Protein: 2g | Carbohydrates: 16g | Fat: 1g | Saturated Fat: 0g
Cholesterol: 8mg | Sodium: 130mg | Fiber: 1g | PCF Ratio: 9-80-10 | Exchange Approx.: 1 Starch

INGREDIENTS | YIELDS 2 LARGE LOAVES; SERVING SIZE: 1 SLICE

2 tablespoons frozen orange juice concentrate

2 tablespoons orange zest

¾ cup pitted, chopped dates

½ cup brown sugar

¼ cup granulated sugar

1 cup plain nonfat yogurt

1 egg

1¼ cups all-purpose flour

¾ cup whole-wheat flour

1 teaspoon baking soda

1 teaspoon baking powder

½ teaspoon salt

1 tablespoon vegetable oil

1 teaspoon vanilla extract

1. Preheat oven to 350°F. Spray 4 mini-loaf pans with nonfat cooking spray.

2. In food processor, process orange juice concentrate, orange zest, dates, sugars, yogurt, and egg until mixed. (This will cut dates into smaller pieces, too.) Add remaining ingredients; pulse until mixed, scraping down side of bowl if necessary.

3. Divide mixture between the pans. Spread the mixture so each pan has an even layer. Bake for 15–20 minutes, or until a toothpick inserted into center of loaf comes out clean.

4. Cool bread in pans on wire rack for 10 minutes. Remove bread to rack and cool to room temperature.

Are Your Eyes Bigger Than Your Stomach?

Use mini-loaf pans. It's much easier to arrive at the number of servings in the form of a full slice when you use smaller loaf pans. There's a psychological advantage to getting a full rather than half slice.

CHAPTER 14

Desserts

Date-Nut Roll

PER SERVING: Calories: 103 | Protein: 2g | Carbohydrates: 18g | Fat: 3g | Saturated Fat: 1g
Cholesterol: 0mg | Sodium: 95mg | Fiber: 1g | PCF Ratio: 7-66-27 | Exchange Approx.: 1 Fat, ½ Starch, ½ Fruit

INGREDIENTS | SERVES 12

12 graham crackers
¼ cup finely chopped walnuts
12 dates, chopped
¼ cup Mock Whipped Cream (page 229)

1. Place graham crackers in plastic bag; use rolling pin to crush or process into crumbs in food processor. Mix crumbs with chopped walnuts and dates. Gently fold in Mock Whipped Cream.

2. Turn mixture out onto a piece of aluminum foil (if you plan to freeze it) or onto plastic wrap (if you'll only be chilling it until you're ready to serve it). Shape into a log; wrap securely in foil or plastic wrap. Chill for at least 4 hours before serving. Cut into 12 slices.

Chocolate Cheesecake Mousse

PER SERVING: Calories: 83 | Protein: 3g | Carbohydrates: 7g | Fat: 5g | Saturated Fat: 2g
Cholesterol: 9mg | Sodium: 47mg | Fiber: 0g | PCF Ratio: 13-32-55 | Exchange Approx.: ½ Skim Milk, 1 Fat

INGREDIENTS | SERVES 4

1 tablespoon semisweet chocolate chips
¾ cup Mock Whipped Cream (page 229)
1 ounce cream cheese
1½ teaspoons cocoa
1 teaspoon vanilla

1. Put chocolate chips and 1 tablespoon of Mock Whipped Cream in microwave-safe bowl; microwave on high for 15 seconds.

2. Add cream cheese; microwave on high for another 15 seconds. Whip mixture until well blended and chocolate chips are melted.

3. Stir in cocoa and vanilla; fold in remaining Mock Whipped Cream. Chill until ready to serve.

Raspberry Yogurt Delight

PER SERVING: Calories: 121 | Protein: 6g | Carbohydrates: 18g | Fat: 3g | Saturated Fat: 2g
Cholesterol: 12mg | Sodium: 74mg | Fiber: 1g | PCF Ratio: 19-59-22 | Exchange Approx.: 1 Milk, ½ Fat

INGREDIENTS | SERVES 4; SERVING SIZE: ½ CUP

1½ cups plain nonfat yogurt
2 tablespoons Splenda granular
4 tablespoons heavy cream
1 tablespoon Splenda granular
¼ cup Raspberry Sauce (below)

1. Combine yogurt and 2 tablespoons Splenda granular in bowl; chill in refrigerator.

2. In separate bowl, whip heavy cream until moderately stiff; stir in 1 tablespoon Splenda granular.

3. To make dessert: Gently fold cream into yogurt. Spoon mixture into 4 dessert or parfait cups. Swirl 1 tablespoon prepared Raspberry Sauce into each cup and serve.

Raspberry Sauce

PER SERVING: Calories: 38 | Protein: 1g | Carbohydrates: 9g | Fat: 0g | Saturated Fat: 0g
Cholesterol: 0mg | Sodium: 1mg | Fiber: 3g | PCF Ratio: 5-89-6 | Exchange Approx.: ½ Fruit

INGREDIENTS | YIELDS 12 SERVINGS; SERVING SIZE: ¼ CUP

4 cups raspberries
2 tablespoons Splenda granular
2 tablespoons honey
1 teaspoon cornstarch
½ tablespoon lemon juice

1. Rinse berries; drain. Put in saucepan; mash.

2. Add Splenda and honey; cook over medium heat until mixture reaches slow boil. Reduce heat; simmer another 10 minutes.

3. Strain berry juice through mesh sieve to remove seeds. Return to saucepan.

4. In separate small bowl, mix cornstarch with lemon juice until dissolved; add to strained berry juice. Bring liquid to a boil, stirring frequently until mixture thickens slightly, about 10 minutes.

5. Cool and store in refrigerator. Use as dessert topping or mixed in yogurt or pudding.

Whipped Lemon Cheesecake Mousse

PER SERVING: Calories: 81 | Protein: 4g | Carbohydrates: 8g | Fat: 4g | Saturated Fat: 3g
Cholesterol: 14mg | Sodium: 65mg | Fiber: 0g | PCF Ratio: 18-38-44 | Exchange Approx.: 1 Skim Milk

INGREDIENTS | SERVES 10; SERVING SIZE: ½ CUP

4 ounces cream cheese, room temperature

1 tablespoon lemon juice

1 teaspoon lemon zest

¼ cup powdered sugar

1 recipe Nonfat Whipped Milk Base (page 230)

In small bowl, combine cream cheese, lemon juice, lemon zest, and sugar; using fork or whisk, beat until well blended. Fold mixture into Whipped Milk Base. Chill for at least 1 hour before serving.

Whipped Mocha Mousse

PER SERVING: Calories: 82 | Protein: 4g | Carbohydrates: 16g | Fat: 1g | Saturated Fat: 0g
Cholesterol: 1mg | Sodium: 37mg | Fiber: 1g | PCF Ratio: 19-77-3 | Exchange Approx.: 1 Skim Milk

INGREDIENTS | SERVES 10; SERVING SIZE: ½ CUP

¼ cup cold water

1 envelope Knox Unflavoured Gelatine

¾ cup hot water

2 teaspoons instant espresso powder

½ cup sugar

¼ cup unsweetened cocoa

1½ teaspoons vanilla extract

1 recipe Nonfat Whipped Milk Base (page 230)

Ground cinnamon (optional)

1. Pour cold water into blender and sprinkle gelatine over it; let stand for 1 minute.

2. Add hot water and instant espresso powder; blend at low speed until gelatine is completely dissolved. Add sugar, cocoa, vanilla, and cinnamon if using; process at high speed until blended. Allow mixture to cool to at least room temperature before folding into Whipped Milk Base. Chill until ready to serve.

Carrot-Fruit Cup

PER SERVING: Calories: 69 | Protein: 1g | Carbohydrates: 18g | Fat: 1g | Saturated Fat: 0g
Cholesterol: 0mg | Sodium: 13mg | Fiber: 4g | PCF Ratio: 4-92-4 | Exchange Approx.: 1 Fruit, ½ Vegetable

INGREDIENTS | SERVES 4; SERVING SIZE: ¾ CUP

1 tablespoon raisins
2 carrots, grated
1 apple, grated
1 tablespoon frozen apple juice concentrate
1 teaspoon cinnamon
Pinch of ginger
1 frozen banana, sliced

1. Soak raisins overnight in little more than enough water to cover.

2. When ready to prepare dessert, drain water from raisins and pour into bowl. Add carrots and apple. Stir in frozen apple juice concentrate and spices until blended. Add banana slices; stir again. Chill until ready to serve.

Fall Fruit with Yogurt Sauce

PER SERVING: Calories: 126 | Protein: 3g | Carbohydrates: 26g | Fat: 3g | Saturated Fat: 1g
Cholesterol: 2mg | Sodium: 48mg | Fiber: 3g | PCF Ratio: 10-72-19 | Exchange Approx.: 1 Fruit, ½ Milk

INGREDIENTS | SERVES 8; SERVING SIZE: ½ CUP

2 cups apples, cubed
1½ cups red seedless grapes, halved
1½ cup pears, cubed
2 teaspoons lemon juice
8 ounces light vanilla yogurt
1 teaspoon lemon juice
1 tablespoon honey
¼ cup walnuts, chopped

1. Combine apples, grapes, and pears in medium bowl. Drizzle 1 teaspoon lemon juice over fruit to prevent turning brown.

2. In small bowl, combine yogurt, 1 teaspoon lemon juice, and honey.

3. Portion ½ cup fruit per serving. Spoon yogurt dressing over fruit and top with chopped walnuts.

Fruit Compote

PER SERVING: Calories: 117 | Protein: 1g | Carbohydrates: 24g | Fat: 2g | Saturated Fat: 1g
Cholesterol: 3mg | Sodium: 29mg | Fiber: 3g | PCF Ratio: 3-80-17 | Exchange Approx.: 1½ Fruits, ½ Fat

INGREDIENTS | SERVES 4; SERVING SIZE: ½ CUP

2 cups apples, chopped

2 tablespoons dried cranberries

6 dried apricots, diced

¼ teaspoon cinnamon

2 tablespoons water

1 tablespoon brandy (optional; if not used, add additional 3 tablespoons water)

1 tablespoon walnuts, finely chopped

1. Combine apples, cranberries, apricots, cinnamon, water, and brandy in small saucepan.

2. Cook over medium heat until apples are softened, about 10 minutes. Remove from heat and cover 5 minutes. Stir in walnuts before serving.

Bubbly Berry Blast

PER SERVING: Calories: 61 | Protein: 2g | Carbohydrates: 13g | Fat: 0g | Saturated Fat: 0g
Cholesterol: 0mg | Sodium: 11mg | Fiber: 1g | PCF Ratio: 15-81-4 | Exchange Approx.: 1 Fruit

INGREDIENTS | SERVES 6; SERVING SIZE: ½ CUP

2 envelopes Knox Unflavoured Gelatine

½ cup frozen unsweetened apple juice concentrate

3 cups (24 ounces) unsweetened sparkling water

1 cup sliced strawberries

1 cup blueberries

1. Mix gelatine and apple juice in small saucepan; stir and let stand for 1 minute. Place mixture over low heat; stir until completely dissolved, about 3 minutes. Cool slightly. (Alternatively, blend gelatine and apple juice in small microwave-safe bowl; let stand 1 minute then microwave on high for 45 seconds; stir until gelatine is completely dissolved.)

2. Stir in sparkling water. Refrigerate until mixture begins to gel or is consistency of unbeaten egg whites when stirred.

3. Fold fruit into partially thickened gelatine mixture. Pour into 6-cup mold. Refrigerate for 4 hours, or until firm.

Faux Chocolate Bavarian Cream

PER SERVING: Calories: 79 | Protein: 7g | Carbohydrates: 13g | Fat: 1g | Saturated Fat: 0g
Cholesterol: 3mg | Sodium: 79mg | Fiber: 1g | PCF Ratio: 33-61-6 | Exchange Approx.: 1 Skim Milk

INGREDIENTS | SERVES 4; SERVING SIZE: ½ CUP

1 envelope Knox Unflavoured Gelatine
⅛ cup cold water
1½ cups skim milk, plus 2 tablespoons
¼ cup nonfat milk powder
2 tablespoons unsweetened cocoa
4 teaspoons sugar
⅛ cup hot water

Tip

This cream is best served right away, but if you have to wait, give it a quick blend just before using to mix in any ingredients that may have separated.

1. While you soak gelatine in cold water (for at least 3 minutes), heat 1½ cups skim milk in saucepan over medium heat just until bubbles begin to form around edges. Turn heat as low as it will go; add milk powder, cocoa, and sugar; stir until they dissolve. Add hot water to gelatine; stir until gelatine dissolves. Add gelatine to milk mixture; stir well. Refrigerate until set, at least 3 hours.

2. Once gelatine has set completely, put in blender with remaining 2 tablespoons of skim milk. Blend until mixture has pudding-like consistency. If necessary, add more milk.

Chocolate Cheesecake Mousse II

PER SERVING: Calories: 104 | Protein: 3g | Carbohydrates: 10g | Fat: 6g | Saturated Fat: 4g
Cholesterol: 11mg | Sodium: 54mg | Fiber: 0g | PCF Ratio: 13-37-51 | Exchange Approx.: 1 Skim Milk, ½ Fat

INGREDIENTS | SERVES 12

4 ounces semisweet chocolate chips
1 recipe Nonfat Whipped Milk Base (page 230)
4 ounces cream cheese, room temperature
1 teaspoon vanilla

Tip

To compensate for differences in whipped textures, this recipe uses more chocolate chips, so the calories per serving are higher than the recipe on page 218.

1. Put chocolate chips in microwave-safe bowl along with ¼ cup Whipped Milk Base. Microwave on high for 20 seconds; beat vigorously with fork or whisk until chocolate is melted and blended in with milk. If necessary, microwave on high for another 5–10 seconds.

2. Cut cream cheese into several pieces, each about 1 tablespoon in size; add to chocolate mixture. Beat vigorously until cream cheese is blended into chocolate.

3. Add vanilla; stir to mix. Pour mixture into remaining Whipped Milk Base; use a spatula to scrape sides of bowl. Chill at least 1 hour before serving.

Chocolate Almond Sauce

PER SERVING: Calories: 36 | Protein: 3g | Carbohydrates: 5g | Fat: 0g | Saturated Fat: 0g
Cholesterol: 1mg | Sodium: 26mg | Fiber: 1g | PCF Ratio: 28-61-11 | Exchange Approx.: ½ Other Carbohydrate

INGREDIENTS | YIELDS 10 SERVINGS;
SERVING SIZE: 2
TABLESPOONS

½ cup cocoa powder
5–6 packets Splenda or other artificial sweetener
8 ounces evaporated skim milk
1 teaspoon almond extract

Something Sweet!
Try this rich sauce over ½ cup of ice cream or a small slice of plain cake. It can be used warm or cold. Mix into 8 ounces skim milk and heat in microwave for hot cocoa. Store sauce in a jar in refrigerator up to 2 weeks.

1. Combine the cocoa and Splenda in small saucepan. Add 1–2 tablespoons evaporated milk and almond extract; stir to make a paste.

2. Add remaining evaporated milk; mix well using whisk. Cook over low heat, stirring constantly, until mixture begins to bubble.

3. Reduce heat and continue cooking for 10 minutes, or until sauce has thickened to consistency of honey.

Peach Bread Pudding

PER SERVING: Calories: 164 | Protein: 7g | Carbohydrates: 23g | Fat: 5g | Saturated Fat: 3g
Cholesterol: 63mg | Sodium: 175mg | Fiber: 2g | PCF Ratio: 16-55-29 | Exchange Approx.: 1 Starch, ½ Fruit, 1 Fat

INGREDIENTS | SERVES 9; SERVING
SIZE: ½ CUP

Nonstick cooking spray
2 cups 1% milk
2 tablespoons butter
2 eggs
⅓ cup egg whites
1 teaspoon vanilla
2 teaspoons cinnamon
⅓ cup Splenda Brown Sugar Blend
6 slices whole-wheat bread, cubed
2 cups peaches, sliced

1. Preheat oven to 350°F. Spray 9" × 9" baking dish with nonstick cooking spray.

2. Heat milk in small saucepan; melt butter in milk. Cool.

3. In medium bowl, beat eggs, egg whites, vanilla, cinnamon, and Splenda.

4. Combine milk and egg mixture.

5. Place cubed bread in baking dish. Place sliced peaches on top of bread cubes. Pour egg mixture over bread and peaches. Bake for 40–45 minutes.

Strawberry-Banana Sherbet

PER SERVING: Calories: 98 | Protein: 4g | Carbohydrates: 22g | Fat: 1g | Saturated Fat: 0g | Cholesterol: 0mg
Sodium: 45mg | Fiber: 2g | PCF Ratio: 13-83-4 | Exchange Approx.: ½ Skim Milk, ½ Fruit, ½ Carbohydrate

INGREDIENTS | SERVES 4; SERVING SIZE: ½ CUP

1⅓ cups strawberry halves

2 tablespoons sugar

1 ripe (but not overly ripe) banana, mashed

1 tablespoon frozen orange juice concentrate

2 tablespoons water

1 tablespoon lemon juice

1 cup 1% milk

2 tablespoons nonfat milk powder

1. Sprinkle sugar over strawberries. Mash strawberries with fork; allow 5 minutes or so for sugar to dissolve and draw juice out of strawberries.

2. Combine all ingredients in blender or food processor; process to desired consistency. (Some people prefer chunks of fruit; others like a smoother sherbet.)

3. Pour mixture into ice-cream maker; freeze according to manufacturer's directions, or pour into ice cube trays or covered container and freeze overnight.

Almond Biscotti

PER SERVING: Calories: 86 | Protein: 2g | Carbohydrates: 13g | Fat: 3g | Saturated Fat: 1g
Cholesterol: 9mg | Sodium: 65mg | Fiber: 0g | PCF Ratio: 8-60-32 | Exchange Approx.: ½ Fat, ½ Starch

INGREDIENTS | YIELDS 42 COOKIES; SERVING SIZE: 1 COOKIE

1 cup sugar

½ cup unsalted butter

1 tablespoon grated orange peel

2 eggs

3½ cups all-purpose flour

1 teaspoon baking powder

½ teaspoon sea salt

⅓ cup ground almonds

1. Preheat oven to 350°F.

2. Beat sugar, butter, orange peel, and eggs in small bowl.

3. Mix together flour, baking powder, and salt in large bowl; stir in egg mixture and almonds.

4. Shape ½ dough at a time into rectangle 10" × 3"; place on ungreased baking sheet. Bake about 20 minutes, or until inserted toothpick comes out clean.

5. Cool on baking sheet for 15 minutes. Cut into ½" slices; place cut-side down on baking sheet. Bake for another 15 minutes, or until crisp and light brown. Cool on a wire rack.

Individual Sponge Cakes

PER SERVING: Calories: 108 | Protein: 3g | Carbohydrates: 21g | Fat: 2g | Saturated Fat: 1g
Cholesterol: 62mg | Sodium: 163mg | Fiber: 1g | PCF Ratio: 12-74-14 | Exchange Approx.: 1½ Starches

INGREDIENTS | YIELDS 12 CAKES;
SERVING SIZE: 1 CAKE

1 cup flour

½ teaspoon salt

1 teaspoon baking powder

3 eggs

¾ cup granulated sugar

1 tablespoon lemon juice

½ teaspoon lemon zest (optional)

6 tablespoons hot milk

Snack Cakes

Use a pastry bag to pump nonfat whipped topping or low-sugar jelly (or a mixture of the two) into the center of the Individual Sponge Cakes, and you have a healthier homemade snack-cake alternative.

1. Preheat oven to 350°F. Mix together flour, salt, and baking powder. In food processor or mixing bowl, beat eggs until fluffy and lemon colored. Add sugar, lemon juice, and lemon zest, if using. Add flour mixture; process only enough to blend. Add milk; process until blended.

2. Pour into a 12-section muffin pan treated with nonstick spray. (Also works well as 24 mini muffins.) If lining muffin pan, use foil liners. Bake for 15 minutes, or until toothpick inserted in center of cake comes out clean. Cakes will be golden brown and firm to the touch. Move cakes to a rack to cool.

Glazed Carrot Cake

PER SERVING: Calories: 149 | Protein: 5g | Carbohydrates: 28g | Fat: 2g | Saturated Fat: 1g
Cholesterol: 42mg | Sodium: 220mg | Fiber: 2g | PCF Ratio: 13-74-13 | Exchange Approx.:
1 Starch, ½ Vegetable, 1 Fruit

INGREDIENTS | SERVES 9

1½ cups unbleached all-purpose flour

1 teaspoon baking powder

1 teaspoon baking soda

1½ teaspoons cinnamon

¼ teaspoon ground cloves

¼ teaspoon ground allspice

⅛ teaspoon ground nutmeg

1 tablespoon sugar

⅛ cup (2 tablespoons) frozen, unsweetened apple juice concentrate

2 eggs

¼ cup water

2 tablespoons ground flaxseed

1 teaspoon vanilla

3 tablespoons nonfat plain yogurt

1 cup canned unsweetened crushed pineapple, ¼ cup of liquid retained

1 cup finely shredded carrots

¼ cup seedless raisins

Glaze

⅛ cup (2 tablespoons) frozen, unsweetened apple juice concentrate

1 tablespoon water

1. Preheat oven to 350°F. Sift together dry ingredients and spices.

2. Using food processor or mixer, blend sugar, apple juice concentrate, and eggs until well mixed. Stir water and flaxseed together in small microwave-safe bowl; microwave on high for 30 seconds, then stir. (Mixture should be consistency of egg whites; if it isn't, microwave at 15-second increments until it is.) Gradually beat into egg mixture, along with vanilla, yogurt, and ¼ cup pineapple liquid.

3. Stir in dry ingredients. Fold in pineapple (drained of any remaining juice), carrots, and raisins.

4. Treat 8" baking pan with nonstick spray. Spoon mixture into pan; bake for 20–25 minutes. Allow cake to cool slightly while you prepare glaze.

5. Mix apple juice concentrate and water until concentrate is melted. (You can microwave the mixture for 15–20 seconds, if necessary.) Spread evenly over cake.

Linzertorte Muffins

PER SERVING: Calories: 147 | Protein: 4g | Carbohydrates: 30g | Fat: 2g | Saturated Fat: 1g
Cholesterol: 16mg | Sodium: 294mg | Fiber: 1g | PCF Ratio: 10-80-10 | Exchange Approx.: 1 Starch, 1 Fruit

INGREDIENTS | YIELDS 12 MUFFINS; SERVING SIZE: 1 MUFFIN

¼ cup ground blanched hazelnuts (filberts)
2 cups unbleached all-purpose flour
2 teaspoons baking powder
½ teaspoon salt
1 teaspoon cinnamon
⅛ teaspoon ground allspice
⅛ teaspoon ground ginger
⅛ cup granulated sugar
¼ cup firmly packed brown sugar
½ cup applesauce
1 egg
1 teaspoon grated lemon peel
½ teaspoon vanilla
1 cup skim milk
12 teaspoons seedless black raspberry jam

1. Preheat oven to 400°F. Spray muffin pan with nonstick spray or use lining cups with cupcake papers.

2. Pulse filberts in food processor until ground. Add all dry ingredients, including spices; pulse until everything is well mixed. Add remaining ingredients except for jam; process to mix. (If you're using a mixer, cream egg, applesauce, and sugars. Mix in milk and vanilla, then add dry ingredients and lemon peel. Fold in nuts.)

3. Spoon a tablespoonful of batter into each of the 12 muffin sections. Top batter with a teaspoonful of seedless black raspberry jam per muffin, being careful no jam touches sides of muffin pan. Evenly divide remaining muffin batter between the 12 muffins, using it to top jam. Gently spread batter to cover jam. Bake 15–20 minutes, or until lightly browned.

Substitution Options

Milk is an easy ingredient to substitute in baking. Fruit juice, rice milk, almond milk (or Ener-G NutQuik), or soy milk (or Ener-G SoyQuik) can be used 1 for 1, although it will alter the nutritional analysis. Keep in mind you can substitute water, but that may produce a blander-tasting baked product.

Mock Whipped Cream

PER SERVING: Calories: 24 | Protein: 1g | Carbohydrates: 2g | Fat: 1g | Saturated Fat: 0g
Cholesterol: 1mg | Sodium: 17mg | Fiber: 0g | PCF Ratio: 21-41-38 | Exchange Approx.: ½ Fat

INGREDIENTS | YIELDS 3½ CUPS; SERVING SIZE: 2 TABLESPOONS

1 envelope Knox Unflavoured Gelatine
¼ cup cold water
½ cup hot water
2 tablespoons almond oil
3 tablespoons powdered sugar
1 teaspoon vanilla
1 cup ice water
1¼ cups nonfat milk powder

Know Your Ingredients

"Gelatine" is the name of the commercial Knox Unflavoured Gelatine product used to make gelatin. Although any unflavored gelatin will work, the nutritional analyses for all recipes are based on the Knox brand.

1. Allow gelatine to soften in cold water; pour into blender. Add hot water; blend for 2 minutes, until gelatin is dissolved.

2. While continuing to blend mixture, gradually add almond oil, powdered sugar, and vanilla. Chill in freezer for 15 minutes, or until mixture is cool but hasn't begun to set.

3. Using hand mixer or whisk, add ice water and nonfat milk powder to a chilled bowl; beat until peaks start to form. Add gelatin mixture to whipped milk; continue to whip for 10 minutes until stiffer peaks begin to form. This whipped topping will keep several days in refrigerator. Whip again to reintroduce more air into topping before serving.

Nonfat Whipped Milk Base

PER RECIPE: Calories: 290 | Carbohydrates: 42g | Protein: 28g | Fat: 1g | Saturated Fat: 0g | Cholesterol: 11mg
Sodium: 310mg | Fiber: 0g | PCF Ratio: 39-59-2 | Exchange Approx.: 2 Skim Milks, 1 Carbohydrate

INGREDIENTS | YIELDS ABOUT 3 CUPS

¼ cup nonfat milk powder
⅛ cup powdered sugar
1 cup chilled skim milk, divided
1½ envelopes Knox Unflavoured Gelatine

Whipping Methods

Because you don't need to whip the Whipped Milk Base until it reaches stiff peaks, you can use a blender or food processor; however, you won't be whipping as much air into the mixture if you do, so the serving sizes will be a bit smaller.

1. In chilled bowl, combine milk powder and sugar; mix until well blended. Pour ¼ cup milk and gelatine into blender; let sit for 1–2 minutes for gelatine to soften.

2. In microwave-safe container, heat remaining milk until it almost reaches boiling point, or 30–45 seconds, on high. Add milk to blender with gelatine; blend 2 minutes, or until gelatine is completely dissolved. Chill for 15 minutes, or until mixture is cool but gelatine hasn't yet begun to set.

3. Using hand mixer or whisk, beat until doubled in size. (It won't form stiff peaks like whipped cream; however, you'll notice it will get creamier in color.) Chill until ready to use in desserts. If necessary, whip again immediately prior to folding in other ingredients.

Key Lime Pie

PER SERVING: Calories: 203 | Protein: 4g | Carbohydrates: 29g | Fat: 8g | Saturated Fat: 4g | Cholesterol: 20mg
Sodium: 331mg | Fiber: 1g | PCF Ratio: 8-57-35 | Exchange Approx.: 1½ Starches, 1½ Fats

INGREDIENTS | SERVES 10; SERVING SIZE: 1 SLICE

1 cup graham cracker crumbs

1 tablespoon Splenda granular

2 tablespoons butter

½ teaspoon lime zest

½ cup Splenda granular

6 ounces low fat (Neufchatel) cream cheese

1 package instant sugar-free vanilla pudding mix

½ cup 1% milk

1 cup key lime juice (5–6 limes)

1 tablespoon Knox Unflavoured Gelatine

1. Prepare graham cracker crust: Combine graham crumbs and 1 tablespoon Splenda. Add melted butter; mix well. Press crumbs into 9" pie plate with help of flat surface such as bottom of glass. Bake in 350°F oven for 10 minutes; remove from oven and cool.

2. In mixer or food processor, combine lime zest and ½ cup Splenda. Add cream cheese; process for 30 seconds. Add pudding mix and milk; blend well.

3. Pour ¼ cup lime juice into small measuring cup or bowl; heat in microwave for 1 minute. Add gelatine to heated juice; dissolve completely.

4. Mix dissolved gelatine in rest of lime juice. Turn on mixer or food processor; pour lime juice into mixture slowly. Process until all ingredients are well combined.

5. Pour filling into pie shell; refrigerate for 3–4 hours before serving. If desired, top with Mock Whipped Cream (page 229).

Strawberry Ricotta Pie

PER SERVING: Calories: 238 | Protein: 10g | Carbohydrates: 27g | Fat: 10g | Saturated Fat: 5g | Cholesterol: 86mg
Sodium: 183mg | Fiber: 1g | PCF Ratio: 18-45-37 | Exchange Approx.: 1 Starch, 1 Lean Meat, 2 Fats

INGREDIENTS | SERVES 8; SERVING SIZE: 1 SLICE

2 cups part-skim ricotta cheese

1 cup graham cracker crumbs

1 tablespoon Splenda granular

2 tablespoons butter

2 eggs, separated

1 teaspoon lemon extract

2 tablespoons honey

¼ cup Splenda granular

¼ cup egg whites

¼ teaspoon cream of tartar

2 cups strawberries, sliced

1 tablespoon cornstarch

2 tablespoons Splenda granular

1 tablespoon lemon juice

1 teaspoon balsamic vinegar

1. Place ricotta cheese in fine mesh strainer lined with coffee filter; allow excess water to drain from cheese for 2–3 hours.

2. Prepare graham cracker crust: Combine graham crumbs and 1 tablespoon Splenda. Add melted butter; mix well. Press crumbs into 9" pie plate with help of flat surface such as bottom of glass. Bake in 350°F oven for 10 minutes; remove from oven and cool.

3. Prepare pie filling: In medium bowl, mix ricotta cheese, egg yolks, lemon extract, honey, and ¼ cup Splenda.

4. In mixer bowl, beat egg whites (2 separated plus ¼ cup additional egg whites) with cream of tartar until soft peaks begin to form. Gently fold egg whites into ricotta mixture. Turn into pie shell; bake at 350°F for 45 minutes, or until mixture is set and top is golden brown. Remove to wire rack and cool completely.

5. Prepare glaze: In medium saucepan, combine strawberries, cornstarch, and Splenda until dry ingredients have coated strawberries. Add lemon juice and balsamic vinegar; cook over medium heat, stirring constantly. Cook mixture for 5–7 minutes, or until cornstarch liquid is clear and gently bubbling. Cool.

6. Spread cooled strawberry glaze on top of cooled pie. Chill until ready to serve.

Summer Fruit Cobbler

PER SERVING: Calories: 152 | Protein: 3g | Carbohydrates: 26g | Fat: 5g | Saturated Fat: 0g | Cholesterol: 0mg
Sodium: 248mg | Fiber: 4g | PCF Ratio: 8-65-27 | Exchange Approx.: ½ Starch, ½ Fruit, 1 Fat

INGREDIENTS | SERVES 8; SERVING SIZE: ½ CUP

Nonstick cooking spray
1½ cups raspberries
1½ cups peaches, peeled and sliced
1 cup strawberries, sliced
¼ cup sugar
1 tablespoon Splenda
2 tablespoons whole-wheat pastry flour
1 teaspoon cinnamon
¾ cup whole-wheat pastry flour
1 tablespoon sugar
1½ teaspoons baking powder
½ teaspoon salt
2½ tablespoons canola oil
2 tablespoons milk
2 tablespoons egg whites

1. Preheat oven to 350°F. Spray 9" × 9" square baking pan with nonstick cooking spray. Put fruit in bottom of baking dish.

2. In small bowl, mix sugar, Splenda, 2 tablespoons flour, and cinnamon; sprinkle evenly over fruit.

3. In small bowl, sift together ¾ cup flour, 1 tablespoon sugar, baking powder, and salt. Add oil, milk, and egg whites; stir quickly until just mixed.

4. Drop dough by spoonfuls over fruit. If desired, loosely spread dough over fruit. Bake for 25–30 minutes, until dough is golden brown.

Fun Fruits

Any combination of fresh fruit will work well with this recipe. You will need a total of 4 cups of fruit. Fruit suggestions include blueberries, blackberries, peaches, mangoes, or plums. Keep in mind that calories will vary somewhat with different fruit combinations.

Baked Pear Crisp

PER SERVING: Calories: 200 | Protein: 2g | Carbohydrates: 42g | Fat: 4g | Saturated Fat: 2g | Cholesterol: 8mg
Sodium: 53mg | Fiber: 3g | PCF Ratio: 3-82-15 | Exchange Approx.: 1 Fruit, 1 Fat, 1 Starch

INGREDIENTS | SERVES 4; SERVING SIZE: ½ CUP

2 pears
2 tablespoons frozen unsweetened pineapple juice concentrate
1 teaspoon vanilla extract
1 teaspoon rum
1 tablespoon butter
⅛ cup Ener-G Brown Rice Flour
⅓ cup firmly packed brown sugar
½ cup oat bran flakes

1. Preheat oven to 375°F. Treat 9" × 13" baking dish or large flat casserole dish with nonstick cooking spray. Core and cut up pears; place in baking dish. (Except for any bruised spots, it's okay to leave skins on.)

2. In glass measuring cup, microwave frozen juice concentrate for 1 minute. Stir in vanilla and rum; pour over pears.

3. Using same measuring cup, microwave butter 30–40 seconds, until melted; set aside.

4. Toss remaining ingredients in bowl, being careful not to crush cereal. Spread uniformly over pears; dribble melted butter over top. Bake for 35 minutes, or until mixture is bubbling and top is just beginning to brown. Serve hot or cold.

Baked Pumpkin Custard

PER SERVING: Calories: 130 | Protein: 7g | Carbohydrates: 23g | Fat: 2g | Saturated Fat: 1g | Cholesterol: 63mg
Sodium: 89mg | Fiber: 2g | PCF Ratio: 20-68-12 | Exchange Approx.: 1 Milk, 1 Vegetable, ½ Fat

INGREDIENTS | SERVES 6; SERVING SIZE: ½ CUP

2 cups solid pack or mashed cooked pumpkin

¼ cup sugar

⅓ cup Splenda granular

2 teaspoons cinnamon

½ teaspoon ginger

⅛ teaspoon cloves

2 eggs, slightly beaten

¼ cup egg whites

12 ounces evaporated skim milk

Pumpkin Pie

If using this recipe for pumpkin pie, pour filling in prepared pie shell and bake in a 350°F oven for 40–45 minutes, or until filling is set. The nutrition information per serving is: Calories: 244; Protein: 8g; Fat: 9g; Saturated fat: 3g; Cholesterol: 63mg; Carbohydrate: 33g; Sodium: 206mg; PCF ratio: 13-33-5; Exchange Approx.: 1 Starch, 1 Milk, 1 Vegetable, 3 Fats.

1. Preheat oven to 350°F.

2. Mix together pumpkin, sugar, Splenda, cinnamon, ginger, and cloves. Add eggs, egg whites, and evaporated milk; whisk until well blended.

3. Pour into 6 custard cups or 1½-quart casserole dish. Set cups or casserole in large baking pan; put pan on rack in oven and pour hot water into pan to within ½" of top of custard.

4. Bake in custard cups for 40–45 minutes, 1½-quart casserole for 60–70 minutes, until knife inserted in center comes out clean. Remove immediately from hot water. Serve warm or chilled.

Strawberry Rhubarb Cobbler

PER SERVING: Calories: 138 | Protein: 3g | Carbohydrates: 27g | Fat: 3g | Saturated Fat: 0g | Cholesterol: 7mg
Sodium: 223mg | Fiber: 3g | PCF Ratio: 7-76-17 | Exchange Approx.: ½ Starch, ½ Fruit, ½ Fat

INGREDIENTS | SERVES 9; SERVING SIZE: ½ CUP

Nonstick cooking spray
4 cups rhubarb, chopped
2 cups strawberries, thickly sliced
¼ teaspoon lemon zest
⅓ cup sugar
¼ cup Splenda granular
2 tablespoons cornstarch
2 tablespoons water
¾ cup whole-wheat pastry flour
1 tablespoon sugar
¼ teaspoon ginger
1½ teaspoons baking powder
½ teaspoon salt
2½ tablespoons canola oil
2 tablespoons milk
2 tablespoons egg whites

1. Preheat oven to 375°F. Spray 8" × 8" baking dish with nonstick cooking spray.

2. In mixing bowl, combine rhubarb, strawberries, lemon zest, sugar, and Splenda. Dissolve cornstarch in water. Pour over fruit; stir to coat. Place in prepared baking dish; set aside.

3. In small bowl, sift together flour, sugar, ginger, baking powder, and salt. Add oil, milk, and egg whites; stir quickly until just mixed.

4. Drop dough by spoonfuls over fruit. If desired, loosely spread dough over fruit. Bake for 25–30 minutes, until dough is golden brown.

Cranberry Pecan Biscotti

PER SERVING: Calories: 98 | Protein: 3g | Carbohydrates: 15g | Fat: 3g | Saturated Fat: 1g | Cholesterol: 20mg
Sodium: 39mg | Fiber: 2g | PCF Ratio: 10-59-3 | Exchange Approx.: 1 Starch, ½ Fat

INGREDIENTS | YIELDS 30 BISCOTTI;
SERVING SIZE: 1
BISCOTTI

4 tablespoons sweet butter, softened
½ cup sugar
½ cup Splenda granular
2 eggs
½ cup egg whites
1 teaspoon vanilla extract
1 teaspoon lemon zest
2½ cups all purpose flour
⅛ teaspoon salt
½ teaspoon baking powder
½ cup pecans, chopped
½ cup dried cranberries

1. Preheat oven to 350°F. In medium bowl, beat butter, sugar, Splenda, eggs, egg whites, vanilla, and lemon zest until smooth.

2. In separate bowl, sift flour, salt, and baking powder. Add dry ingredients to liquid ingredients; mix well. Add pecans and cranberries. Chill dough for 1–2 hours, which makes it easier to handle.

3. Divide dough in ½; shape each ½ into slightly flattened 3" × 9" loaf. Place loaves on greased cookie sheet; bake for 25 minutes.

4. Remove from oven; when cooled enough to handle, cut into ½" slices. Lay out slices on cookie sheet and return to oven for 20 minutes until toasted on bottom.

5. Remove from oven; turn over and bake for 15 minutes until other side is toasted as well. Remove from oven and cool on wire rack.

Bananas Foster

PER SERVING: Calories: 220 | Protein: 2g | Carbohydrates: 51g | Fat: 1g | Saturated Fat: 0g
Cholesterol: 0mg | Sodium: 43mg | Fiber: 4g | PCF Ratio: 4-92-4 | Exchange Approx.: 2½ Fruits, 1 Skim Milk

INGREDIENTS | SERVES 4

4 bananas, sliced

¼ cup apple juice concentrate

Grated zest of 1 orange

¼ cup fresh orange juice

1 tablespoon ground cinnamon

12 ounces nonfat frozen vanilla yogurt

Know Your Ingredients

Overripe bananas are higher in sugar and can adversely affect blood glucose levels. Freeze bananas in skins until ready to use. Doing so makes them perfect additions for fruit smoothies or fruit cups. Remove from freezer and run a little water over peel to remove any frost. Peel using a paring knife and slice according to recipe directions. Frozen bananas can be added directly to smoothies and other recipes.

1. Combine all ingredients except yogurt in nonstick skillet. Bring to a boil; cook until bananas are tender.

2. Put 3 ounces frozen yogurt in each dessert bowl or stemmed glass; spoon heated banana sauce over top.

Raspberry Trifle

PER SERVING: Calories: 211 | Protein: 7g | Carbohydrates: 34g | Fat: 5g | Saturated Fat: 1g | Cholesterol: 62mg
Sodium: 464mg | Fiber: 4g | PCF Ratio: 15-64-21 | Exchange Approx.: ½ Milk, ½ Starch, ½ Fruit, 1 Fat

INGREDIENTS | SERVES 4

4 Individual Sponge Cakes (page 226)
1 (1.3-ounce) package vanilla sugar-free instant pudding mix
2 cups 1% milk, for pudding
1 teaspoon almond extract
2 packets Splenda
1½ cups fresh raspberries

Trifle Toppings

If desired, top each serving with tablespoon of Mock Cream (page 183) or Raspberry Sauce (page 219). Either will add calories to the dessert, so plan accordingly. One tablespoon Mock Whipped Cream adds 24 calories and 1 tablespoon Raspberry Sauce adds 38 extra calories.

1. Slice each sponge cake into 4 small slices.

2. Follow package directions for pudding mix. Add almond extract to pudding, while mixing.

3. Add Splenda to fresh raspberries; mix gently until Splenda has dissolved.

4. Assemble trifle: Arrange ½ of cake slices in circle in bottom of small glass bowl or dish. (You can also use individual glass goblets and follow same procedure.) Place ½ of raspberries over top of cakes. Spread ½ of pudding over fruit, leaving ½" border all around. Repeat layer of cake, raspberries, and pudding. Wrap bowl in plastic wrap; refrigerate for at least 6 hours.

Apple Cookies with a Kick

PER SERVING: Calories: 64 | Protein: 2g | Carbohydrates: 12g | Fat: 1g | Saturated Fat: 0g
Cholesterol: 0mg | Sodium: 67mg | Fiber: 1g | PCF Ratio: 12-71-17 | Exchange Approx.: 1 Fruit

INGREDIENTS | YIELDS 24 COOKIES; SERVING SIZE: 1 COOKIE

1 tablespoon ground flaxseed
¼ cup water
¼ cup firmly packed brown sugar
⅛ cup granulated sugar
¾ cup cooked pinto beans, drained
⅓ cup unsweetened applesauce
2 teaspoons baking powder
⅛ teaspoon sea salt
1 teaspoon ground cinnamon
½ teaspoon ground nutmeg
¼ teaspoon ground cloves
¼ teaspoon ground allspice
1 cup Vita-Spelt white spelt flour
1 medium-sized Golden Delicious apple
1 cup dried sunflower seed kernels (unroasted, unsalted)

1. Preheat oven to 350°F.

2. Put flaxseed and water in microwave-safe container; microwave on high for 15 seconds, or until mixture thickens and has consistency of egg whites. Add flaxseed mixture, sugars, beans, and applesauce to mixing bowl; mix well.

3. Sift dry ingredients together; fold into bean mixture. (Do not overmix; this will cause muffins to become tough.)

4. Peel and chop apple; fold into batter with sunflower seeds.

5. Drop by teaspoonful onto baking sheet treated with nonstick spray; bake for 12–18 minutes.

Creative Substitutions

Adding nuts and, of all things, beans to dessert recipes increases the amount of protein and fiber. Just because it's dessert doesn't mean it has to be all empty calories.

Pineapple Upside-Down Cake

PER SERVING: Calories: 138 | Protein: 3g | Carbohydrates: 32g | Fat: 0g | Saturated Fat: 0g
Cholesterol: 0g | Sodium: 83g | Fiber: 1mg | PCF Ratio: 7-92-1 | Exchange Approx.: 1 Starch, 1 Fruit

INGREDIENTS | SERVES 8

1 tablespoon brown sugar

1 (8¼-ounce) can unsweetened crushed pineapple in juice (drained, juice reserved)

1 envelope Knox Unflavoured Gelatine

2 eggs

1 egg white

¾ cup granulated sugar

1 teaspoon vanilla

¾ cup all-purpose flour

1 teaspoon baking powder

¼ teaspoon salt

1. Preheat oven to 375°F. Line 9" × 1½" round baking pan with waxed paper and spray with nonstick cooking spray. Sprinkle brown sugar on waxed paper. Spread crushed pineapple evenly in bottom of pan; sprinkle gelatine over top.

2. In large bowl, beat eggs and egg white until very thick. Gradually beat in granulated sugar. Add enough water to reserved pineapple juice to measure ⅓ cup; beat into egg mixture along with vanilla.

3. In separate bowl, mix flour, baking powder, and salt; gradually add to egg mixture, beating until batter is smooth. Pour into pan. Bake about 25–30 minutes, or until inserted toothpick comes out clean. Immediately loosen cake from edge of pan with knife; invert pan on plate. Carefully remove waxed paper; slice into 8 pieces.

Whole-Grain Maple-Walnut Bread Pudding

PER SERVING: Calories: 140 | Protein: 6g | Carbohydrates: 18g | Fat: 5g | Saturated Fat: 1g | Cholesterol: 55mg
Sodium: 103mg | Fiber: 1g | PCF Ratio: 16-51-33 | Exchange Approx.: 1 Starch, 1 Fat, ½ Misc. Carbohydrate

INGREDIENTS | SERVES 8

1 cup skim milk

⅜ cup dry nonfat milk powder

2 teaspoons unsalted butter

2 eggs

1 teaspoon vanilla

3 tablespoons maple syrup

1 tablespoon brown sugar

Pinch of sea salt (optional)

4 ounces 7-Grain Bread (4 thick slices with crusts removed; page 203)

¼ cup chopped walnuts

1. Preheat oven to 350°F.

2. Put milk, milk powder, butter, eggs, vanilla, syrup, brown sugar, and salt, if using, in food processor or blender; process until mixed.

3. Tear crustless bread into pieces; place in mixing bowl. Pour blended milk mixture over bread and add chopped walnuts; toss to mix.

4. Pour mixture into nonstick cake pan. Bake for 20 minutes, or until egg is set. Cut into 8 pie-shaped wedges. Serve warm or chilled.

CHAPTER 15

Snacks and Beverages

Tortilla Chips

PER SERVING: Calories: 81 | Protein: 1g | Carbohydrates: 15g | Fat: 5g | Saturated Fat: 1g
Cholesterol: 0mg | Sodium: 30mg | Fiber: 1g | PCF Ratio: 5-54-41 | Exchange Approx.: 1 Starch, ½ Fat

INGREDIENTS | SERVES 1

1 nonfat corn tortilla
Olive oil
Sea salt, to taste (optional)
Seasoning blend of your choice, to taste

Tip

When you buy tortillas, look for a brand made with only cornmeal, water, and lime juice. Nutritional analysis and exchange approximations will depend on the brand of tortillas and amount of oil you use.

1. Preheat oven to 400°F. Spray both sides of tortilla with olive oil. Season lightly with sea salt or any seasoning blend.

2. Bake tortilla on cookie sheet until crisp and beginning to brown, 2–5 minutes, depending on thickness of tortilla. Break tortilla into large pieces.

Zucchini with Cheese Spread

PER SERVING: Calories: 38 | Protein: 4g | Carbohydrates: 4g | Fat: 0g | Saturated Fat: 0g
Cholesterol: 2mg | Sodium: 140mg | Fiber: 2g | PCF Ratio: 42-43-15 | Exchange Approx.: 1 Vegetable, ½ Fat

INGREDIENTS | SERVES 8;
SERVING SIZE: 1
TABLESPOON

1 large green zucchini
⅓ cup softened fat-free cream cheese
¼ cup finely chopped red bell pepper
2 teaspoons dried parsley
¼ teaspoon onion powder
¼ teaspoon dried Italian seasoning
2 drops red pepper sauce
1 green onion, thinly sliced

1. Peel zucchini; cut into ¼" slices. Mix remaining ingredients except green onion until well blended.

2. Spread 1–2 teaspoons of cream cheese mixture onto each slice of zucchini; place on serving platter. Sprinkle with green onion; cover and refrigerate for 1 hour, or until firm.

Toasted Pumpkin Seeds

PER SERVING, without salt: Calories: 202 | Protein: 9g | Carbohydrates: 6g | Fat: 18g | Saturated Fat: 3g
Cholesterol: 0mg | Sodium: 6mg | Fiber: 1g | PCF Ratio: 16-11-73 | Exchange Approx.: 1 Lean Meat, 3 Fats

INGREDIENTS | **SERVES 8; SERVING SIZE: ¼ CUP**

2 cups pumpkin seeds, scooped from fresh pumpkin

1 tablespoon olive, peanut, or canola oil

Sea salt (optional)

1. Rinse pumpkin seeds, removing all pulp and strings; spread seeds in single layer on large baking sheet. Let air dry for at least 3 hours.

2. Preheat oven to 375°F. Drizzle oil over seeds and lightly sprinkle with salt, if using. (Alternative method would be to put dried pumpkin seeds in a plastic bag and add oil. Seal bag; toss to mix.) Toss; spread out in single layer.

3. Bake for 15 to 20 minutes, until lightly browned and toasted. Stir the seeds occasionally during the baking to allow for even browning. Remove hulls to eat.

Black Olive Mock Caviar

PER SERVING: Calories: 21 | Protein: 0g | Carbohydrates: 1g | Fat: 2g | Saturated Fat: 0g | Cholesterol: 0mg
Sodium: 85mg | Fiber: 0g | PCF Ratio: 3-25-73 | Exchange Approx.: 1 Free Condiment or ½ Fat

INGREDIENTS | **YIELDS 1¼ CUPS; SERVING SIZE: 1 TABLESPOON**

1 (5¾-ounce) can chopped black olives

1 (4-ounce) can chopped green chili peppers

1 cup diced fresh or canned (no salt added) tomato

2 tablespoons chopped green onions

1 clove garlic, minced

1 tablespoon extra-virgin olive oil

1 teaspoon red wine vinegar

Pinch of sugar

½ teaspoon freshly ground black pepper

In medium-sized mixing bowl, mix together all ingredients. Cover; chill overnight. Serve cold or at room temperature.

Creamy Fruit Cup

PER SERVING, without additional applesauce or jelly: Calories: 128 | Protein: 7g | Carbohydrates: 26g
Fat: 1g | Saturated Fat: 0g | Cholesterol: 0mg | Sodium: 89mg | Fiber: 2g | PCF Ratio: 19-77-3 | Exchange
Approx.: ½ Skim Milk, 1½ Fruits

INGREDIENTS | SERVES 1

4 ounces (half small container) nonfat plain yogurt

1 tablespoon unsweetened applesauce

1 teaspoon lemon juice

½ cup cubed fresh or frozen cantaloupe

¼ cup cubed or sliced apple

6 seedless red or green grapes

Lemon zest (optional)

1. Mix together yogurt, applesauce, and lemon juice; drizzle over mixed fruit. (If you prefer a sweeter dressing, you can add another tablespoon of applesauce or blend in 2 teaspoons of low-sugar apple jelly without increasing the number of fruit exchanges; adjust calorie count accordingly.)

2. Sprinkle lemon zest over top of dressing.

Just Juice?

Fruit and fruit juice provide healthy nutrients, and, in most cases, fiber, too. That's the good news. The downside is they also convert quickly to glucose. For that reason, many people can only consume them as part of a meal, rather than alone as a snack.

Sparkling Fruited Iced Tea

PER SERVING: Calories: 62 | Protein: 0g | Carbohydrates: 16g | Fat: 0g | Saturated Fat: 0g
Cholesterol: 0mg | Sodium: 12mg | Fiber: 0g | PCF Ratio: 3-97-1 | Exchange Approx.: 1 Fruit

INGREDIENTS | SERVES 4

3 cups decaffeinated tea

1 cup unsweetened orange juice

4 teaspoons fresh lemon juice

1 (12-ounce) can carbonated ginger ale

Seltzer water, club soda, or other unsweetened carbonated water

1. In pitcher, mix together tea, orange juice, and lemon juice. In tall iced-tea glasses (16- to 20-ounce size), place 4 or 5 ice cubes.

2. Pour tea and juice mixture over ice; evenly divide ginger ale between glasses.

3. Add carbonated water to finish filling glasses; stir to mix. Serve.

Ginger Lime Iced Tea

PER SERVING: Calories: 23 | Protein: 0g | Carbohydrates: 6g | Fat: 0g | Saturated Fat: 0g | Cholesterol: 0mg Sodium: 0mg | Fiber: 0g | PCF Ratio: 1-99-0 | Exchange Approx.: ½ Misc. Carbohydrate

INGREDIENTS | SERVES 6

6 cups boiling water

4 green tea bags

2 tablespoons honey

1 tablespoon lime juice

1 tablespoon coarsely chopped crystallized ginger

1. In ceramic or glass container, pour boiling water over tea bags, honey, lime juice, and ginger; cover and allow to steep for 5 minutes. Stir until honey is dissolved.

2. Remove teabags and ginger. Chill in refrigerator and serve over ice. (May also be served hot.)

Orange-Pineapple Froth

PER SERVING: Calories: 153 | Protein: 9g | Carbohydrates: 27g | Fat: 1g | Saturated Fat: 0g | Cholesterol: 5mg Sodium: 129mg | Fiber: 0g | PCF Ratio: 24-73-3 | Exchange Approx.: 2 Fruits, 1 Skim Milk

INGREDIENTS | SERVES 1

1 tablespoon frozen orange juice concentrate

1 tablespoon frozen pineapple juice concentrate

1 cup skim milk

½ cup chilled water

½ teaspoon vanilla

Combine all ingredients in blender; process until mixed. Serve in chilled glass.

Minted Raspberry Lemonade

PER SERVING: Calories: 19 | Protein: 0g | Carbohydrates: 6g | Fat: 0g | Saturated Fat: 0g
Cholesterol: 0mg | Sodium: 4mg | Fiber: 1g | PCF Ratio: 5-93-2 | Exchange Approx.: ½ Fruit

INGREDIENTS | SERVES 8

½ cup raspberries

1½ cups lemon juice

8 packets sweetener, or to taste

6 cups water

1 tablespoon finely chopped fresh mint, or 1 teaspoon dried mint

1. Mash raspberries; press through fine-mesh sieve to remove seeds.

2. Add raspberries, lemon juice, sweetener, water, and mint to 2-quart pitcher; stir. Serve chilled over ice.

Bubbly Touch-of-Fruit Taste Drink

Another soft drink option is to pour a cup of chilled, unsweetened club soda or seltzer over fresh or frozen fruit. The fruit imparts subtle flavor and sweetness to the beverage, and when the drink is gone, you can eat the fruit for dessert. The nutritional analysis depends on the chosen fruit, but for any choice, Exchange Approx.: ½ Fruit.

Iced Ginger-Orange Green Tea

PER SERVING: Calories: 62 | Protein: 1g | Carbohydrates: 14g | Fat: 0g | Saturated Fat: 0g
Cholesterol: 0mg | Sodium: 9mg | Fiber: 0g | PCF Ratio: 6-90-4 | Exchange Approx.: 1 Fruit

INGREDIENTS | SERVES 4

2 cups water

1 tablespoon coarsely chopped crystallized ginger

2 (1") pieces orange peel

4 green tea bags

2 cups orange juice, chilled

Monitor Your Exchanges

If you add additional sweetener to any of the tea recipes, be sure to include that exchange list choice as well, if applicable.

1. In medium saucepan, bring water to boil.

2. In ceramic container, pour boiling water over ginger and orange peel. Add tea bags; cover and steep for 5 minutes.

3. Remove tea bags, ginger, and orange peel; add orange juice and stir. Put ice cubes in 4 glasses; pour orange juice–tea blend over ice and serve.

Almond-Flavored Hot Cocoa

PER SERVING: Calories: 126 | Protein: 9g | Carbohydrates: 15g | Fat: 3g | Saturated Fat: 2g
Cholesterol: 12mg | Sodium: 107mg | Fiber: 1g | PCF Ratio: 30-49-21 | Exchange Approx.: 1 Skim Milk

INGREDIENTS | SERVES 1

1 tablespoon cocoa powder
1 packet artificial sweetener
1 cup skim milk
¼ teaspoon almond extract

1. Mix cocoa powder, sweetener, 1 tablespoon of milk, and almond extract in mug and make a paste.

2. Add remaining milk to paste; mix well. Microwave on high for 1½–2 minutes, or until milk is heated.

Hot Spiced Tea

PER SERVING: Calories: 8 | Protein: 0g | Carbohydrates: 2g | Fat: 0g | Saturated Fat: 0g
Cholesterol: 0mg | Sodium: 3mg | Fiber: 0g | PCF Ratio: 5-93-2 | Exchange Approx.: ½ Free

INGREDIENTS | SERVES 4

2 tea bags
14 whole cloves
1 cinnamon stick
1 strip (about 3") fresh orange peel
2 cups boiling water
¼ cup orange juice
1½ tablespoons lemon juice

1. Put tea bags, spices, and orange peel in ceramic or glass container; pour boiling water over. Cover and allow to steep for 5 minutes.

2. Strain; stir in orange and lemon juices. Reheat if necessary. You can also chill it and serve over ice for a refreshing iced tea.

Frothy Orange Jewel

PER SERVING: Calories: 135 | Protein: 9g | Carbohydrates: 23g | Fat: 1g | Saturated Fat: 0g | Cholesterol: 5mg
Sodium: 128mg | Fiber: 0g | PCF Ratio: 27-69-4 | Exchange Approx.: 1 Fruit, 1 Skim Milk

INGREDIENTS | SERVES 1

¼ cup fresh orange juice

1 cup skim milk

1½ teaspoons powdered sugar

½ teaspoon vanilla

1–2 ice cubes (optional)

Combine all ingredients in blender; process until mixed. Serve in frosted glass. If you don't have fresh orange juice on hand, you can substitute 1 tablespoon frozen orange juice concentrate and 3 tablespoons of water.

Kiwi-Lime Cooler

PER SERVING: Calories: 135 | Protein: 8g | Carbohydrates: 26g | Fat: 1g | Saturated Fat: 0g
Cholesterol: 2mg | Sodium: 97mg | Fiber: 3g | PCF Ratio: 23-73-5 | Exchange Approx.: 1 Skim Milk, 1 Fruit

INGREDIENTS | SERVES 2

1 cup ice cubes

1 tablespoon lime juice

1 cup light vanilla yogurt

2 ripe kiwi, peeled and sliced

1–2 packets artificial sweetener, or to taste

Combine all ingredients in blender; process until mixed. Serve in chilled glass.

The Chinese Gooseberry

Kiwi is also known as Chinese Gooseberrry. Kiwi is a very nutrient-dense food rich in vitamin C, fiber, and potassium. This versatile little fruit can be used in beverages, salads, salsas, or as a beautiful edible garnish. Native to China, kiwi is now grown in many parts of the world, and is easy to find in grocery stores and produce markets.

Strawberry Cooler

PER SERVING: Calories: 52 | Protein: 1g | Carbohydrates: 13g | Fat: 0g | Saturated Fat: 0g
Cholesterol: 0mg | Sodium: 3mg | Fiber: 2g | PCF Ratio: 4-91-6 | Exchange Approx.: 1 Fruit

INGREDIENTS | SERVES 1

½ cup frozen strawberries
¼ cup apple juice
Sparkling water

In a large tumbler, place frozen strawberries. Pour apple juice over strawberries; finish filling glass with sparkling water. Stir, and serve with an iced-tea spoon.

Nectarine Cocktail

PER SERVING: Calories: 109 | Protein: 5g | Carbohydrates: 21g | Fat: 1g | Saturated Fat: 1g | Cholesterol: 4mg
Sodium: 131mg | Fiber: 1g | PCF Ratio: 17-72-11 | Exchange Approx.: 1 Fruit, ½ Skim Milk

INGREDIENTS | SERVES 4

2 cups buttermilk
2 large chilled nectarines, peeled and cut into pieces
⅛ cup brown sugar

Combine buttermilk, nectarines, and brown sugar in blender; process until nectarines are puréed. Serve in chilled glass.

Snack Mix

PER SERVING, on average: Calories: 125 | Protein: 3g | Carbohydrates: 16g | Fat: 5g
Cholesterol: 4mg | Sodium: 201mg | Fiber: 2g | PCF Ratio: variable | Exchange Approx.: 1 Starch, 1 Fat

INGREDIENTS | SERVES 16; SERVING SIZE: ½ CUP

6 cups mixed cereal (such as a mixture of unsweetened bran, oat, rice, and wheat cereals)

1 cup mini bow-knot pretzels

⅔ cup dry-roasted peanuts

⅛ cup (2 tablespoons) butter, melted

⅛ cup (2 tablespoons) olive, canola, or peanut oil

1 tablespoon Worcestershire sauce (see recipe on page 192)

¼ teaspoon garlic powder

Tabasco sauce or other liquid hot pepper sauce, to taste (optional)

1. Preheat oven to 300°F. In large bowl, combine cereals, pretzels, and peanuts.

2. In another bowl, combine butter, oil, Worcestershire, garlic powder, and Tabasco, if using. Pour over cereal mixture; toss to coat evenly.

3. Spread mixture on large baking sheet; bake for 30–40 minutes, stirring every 10 minutes, until crisp and dry. Cool and store in airtight container. Serve at room temperature.

Tip
The nutritional analysis will depend on the type of fat and cereals used in the recipe, most notably regarding the PCF Ratio.

No-Bake Chocolate–Peanut Butter Oatmeal Cookies

PER SERVING, with granulated sugar: Calories: 87 | Protein: 2g | Carbohydrates: 13g | Fat: 3g | Saturated Fat: 2g
Cholesterol: 5mg | Sodium: 26mg | Fiber: 1g | PCF Ratio: 7-61-32 | Exchange Approx.: ½ Fat, 1 Starch

INGREDIENTS | SERVES 12; SERVING SIZE: 1 COOKIE

2 tablespoons butter

¼ cup cocoa

½ cup granulated sugar

¼ cup Mock Cream (page 183)

Dash of sea salt

1 teaspoon vanilla

1 tablespoon peanut butter

1½ cups oatmeal

1. Add butter to deep, microwave-safe bowl; microwave on high for 20–30 seconds, or until butter is melted.

2. Add cocoa; stir to blend. Stir in sugar, Mock Cream, and salt; microwave on high for 1 minute, 10 seconds to bring to full boil. (Should you need to microwave batter more, do so in 10-second increments. You want a full boil, but because it will continue to cook for a while once it's removed from microwave, heating too long can cause mixture to scorch.)

3. Add vanilla and peanut butter; stir until mixed. Fold in oatmeal. Drop by tablespoonful on waxed paper and allow to cool.

Iced and Spiced Chai-Style Tea

PER SERVING: Calories: 108 | Protein: 4g | Carbohydrates: 23g | Fat: 1g | Saturated Fat: 0g | Cholesterol: 0mg
Sodium: 65mg | Fiber: 0g | PCF Ratio: 14-82-4 | Exchange Approx.: 1 Misc. Carbohydrate, ½ Skim Milk

INGREDIENTS | SERVES 4

2 cups skim milk

¼ cup honey (optional)

½ teaspoon ground cinnamon

¼ teaspoon ground ginger

⅛ teaspoon allspice

4 tea bags

2 cups chilled unflavored, unsweetened carbonated water

1. In medium saucepan, bring milk just to boil. Stir in remaining ingredients except for carbonated water. Reduce heat to low and simmer, uncovered, for 3 minutes.

2. Remove tea bags and strain; chill. Serve over ice, adding an equal amount of carbonated water to each serving.

Tip

Alternative serving suggestion: This tea is also terrific when served warm in mugs; just replace the carbonated water with warm water.

Asian Popcorn

PER SERVING: Calories: 129 | Protein: 3g | Carbohydrates: 26g | Total Fat: 1g | Saturated Fat: 0g | Cholesterol: 0mg
Sodium: 221mg | Fiber: 5g | PCF Ratio: 14-77-9 | Exchange Approx.: 1 Starch, 1 Free Condiment

INGREDIENTS | SERVES 1

4 cups air-popped popcorn

Nonstick or butter-flavored cooking spray

1 teaspoon Bragg's Liquid Aminos, or low-sodium soy sauce

2 teaspoons fresh lemon juice

1 teaspoon five spice powder

¼ teaspoon ground coriander

¼ teaspoon garlic powder

1. Preheat oven to 250°F. Spread popcorn on nonstick cookie sheet; lightly coat with nonstick or butter-flavored cooking spray.

2. Mix together all remaining ingredients. Drizzle over popcorn; lightly toss to coat evenly. Bake for 5 minutes; toss popcorn and rotate pan; bake for an additional 5 minutes. Serve warm.

Keeping Snacks in Stock

Because there are no oils to go rancid, air-popped popcorn will keep for weeks if you store it in an airtight container. Pop a large batch and keep some on hand for later. Flavor it according to your taste, and you'll have a warm, healthy snack.

Fruit Frenzy Sparkler Concentrate

PER SERVING: Calories: 53 | Protein: 1g | Carbohydrates: 13g | Fat: 0g | Saturated Fat: 0g
Cholesterol: 0mg | Sodium: 1mg | Fiber: 1g | PCF Ratio: 5-91-4 | Exchange Approx.: 1 Fruit

INGREDIENTS | SERVES 8

1 cup peeled, seeded, and chopped peach or papaya

1 cup peeled and cubed fresh pineapple

1 teaspoon peeled and grated fresh ginger

1 cup orange juice

1 cup frozen banana slices

Unsweetened club soda, seltzer water, or carbonated water

Place all ingredients except water in food processor; process until smooth. To serve, pour ½ cup concentrate over ice in 12- to 16-ounce glass. Complete filling glass with carbonated water.

Spiced Chai-Style Creamer Mix

PER SERVING: Calories: 86 | Protein: 4g | Carbohydrates: 17g | Fat: 0g | Saturated Fat: 0g | Cholesterol: 0mg
Sodium: 65mg | Fiber: 0g | PCF Ratio: 20-78-2 | Exchange Approx.: 1 Misc. Carbohydrate

INGREDIENTS | YIELDS 15 TEASPOONS; SERVING SIZE: 1 TABLESPOON

½ cup nonfat dry milk

1½ teaspoons cinnamon

¼ teaspoon nutmeg

¼ teaspoon ground cloves

½ teaspoon ginger

¼ teaspoon allspice

¼ cup sugar

Combine all ingredients in lidded jar; shake to mix. Store in a cool, dry place. Because this recipe uses noninstant nonfat milk, it must be stirred into hot liquid. For iced tea, you can mix in "creamer" using a blender.

Pineapple-Banana Blast

PER SERVING: Calories: 109 | Protein: 5g | Carbohydrates: 21g | Fat: 1g | Saturated Fat: 1g
Cholesterol: 4mg | Sodium: 129mg | Fiber: 1g | PCF Ratio: 16-74-10 | Exchange Approx.: 1 Fruit, ½ Skim Milk

INGREDIENTS | SERVES 1

¼ frozen banana, sliced

1 tablespoon frozen pineapple juice concentrate

3 tablespoons water

½ cup buttermilk

Combine all ingredients in blender; process until mixed. Serve in chilled glass.

Chocolate Candy Substitute

PER SERVING: Calories: 11 | Protein: 0g | Carbohydrates: 2g | Fat: 0g | Saturated Fat: 0g | Cholesterol: 0mg
Sodium: 0mg | Fiber: 0g | PCF Ratio: 0-100-0 | Exchange Approx. (for entire recipe, without dry milk): 1 Fruit

INGREDIENTS | YIELDS 15–20 PIECES; SERVING SIZE: 1 PIECE

1 tablespoon cocoa

1 tablespoon sugar

¾ cup fresh pineapple chunks

1–3 teaspoons nonfat dry milk (optional)

Tip

The exchange approximations given for this recipe are for the entire amount; however, it's intended to be used as a way to curb a candy craving. (You grab a frozen chunk from the freezer and eat it like candy.) Discuss this recipe with your dietitian to see how you can fit it into your meal plan.

1. In small bowl, mix cocoa and sugar.

2. Place waxed paper on baking sheet. Dip each piece of pineapple in cocoa-sugar mixture. (The choice whether to coat only 1 side of the pineapple or all sides depends on whether you prefer a dark, bittersweet chocolate taste or a milder one. Add dry milk powder to mixture if you prefer milk chocolate. Place each piece of pineapple on waxed paper–covered baking sheet. Place baking sheet in freezer for several hours.

3. Once pineapple is frozen, layer "candies" on waxed paper in airtight freezer container. Place a piece of aluminum foil over top layer before putting on lid, to prevent freezer burn.

Tangy Limeade

PER SERVING, without salt: Calories: 65 | Protein: 0g | Carbohydrates: 18g | Fat: 0g | Saturated Fat: 0g
Cholesterol: 0mg | Sodium: 1mg | Fiber: 1.41g | PCF Ratio: 2-97-1 | Exchange Approx.: 1 Misc. Carbohydrate

INGREDIENTS | SERVES 8

6 fresh limes
½ cup granulated sugar
2½ cups water
½ teaspoon salt (optional)
12 ice cubes, or 1½ cups cold water

Carbonated Limeade

To make a concentrate that can be stored in refrigerator for up to 3 days, reduce the boiling water to 1 cup. In a glass, combine 3 tablespoons of the concentrate with enough seltzer water or club soda to fill an 8- to 12-ounce glass. Remember that more carbonated water will produce a weaker-tasting beverage. Exchange Approximations: 1 Misc. Carbohydrate, ½ Fruit.

1. Roll limes on cutting board using hard pressure to loosen flesh and release juices. Cut limes in ½ and juice them, minus any seeds and pith. Place rinds in noncorrosive metal or glass container; cover with sugar, and set aside.

2. Bring water to boil; pour over lime juice, rinds, and sugar mixture. Allow to steep for 5–10 minutes, depending on your taste. (2 minutes is sufficient for an intense lime flavor; 10 minutes will have a hint of bitterness. If you prefer a sweeter limeade, omit rinds and steep mixture with juice and pulp.)

3. If you're using optional salt, add it now and stir thoroughly. Strain warm liquid. Add ice cubes; stir until ice is melted. Serve over additional ice cubes.

Peachy Ginger Ale

PER SERVING: Calories: 43 | Protein: 0g | Carbohydrates: 11g | Fat: 0g | Saturated Fat: 0g | Cholesterol: 0mg
Sodium: 3mg | Fiber: 1g | PCF Ratio: 3-97-1 | Exchange Approx.: ½ Fruit, ½ Misc. Carbohydrate

INGREDIENTS | SERVES 4

1 large peach
⅛ cup brown sugar
2 teaspoons minced fresh ginger
⅛ cup water
Unsweetened club soda, seltzer water, or carbonated water

1. Peel peach; cut into 10 slices. Place 8 slices on tray; set in freezer. Put remaining 2 slices of peach in bowl; mash with a fork. Add brown sugar; mash with peach. Set aside.

2. In microwave-safe container, mix ginger with water; microwave on high for 2 minutes. Cover container and allow mixture to steep for 5 minutes. Strain ginger water (to remove the ginger) over peach-brown sugar mixture; stir until brown sugar is completely dissolved.

3. Remove peach slices from freezer; put 2 slices in each of 4 (12-ounce) glasses. Divide ginger-peach mixture between glasses. Pour unsweetened carbonated water over frozen fruit; stir. Serve with an iced-tea spoon.

Powdered Sugar-Coated Cocoa Cookies

PER SERVING, using plums packed in heavy syrup: Calories: 66 | Protein: 1g | Carbohydrates: 14g
Fat: 1g | Saturated Fat: 1g | Cholesterol: 3mg | Sodium: 41mg | Fiber: 1g | PCF Ratio: 5-78-17
Exchange Approx.: 1 Starch

**INGREDIENTS | YIELDS 24 COOKIES;
SERVING SIZE: 1 COOKIE**

1 tablespoon ground flaxseed
2 tablespoons water or plum juice
2 tablespoons unsalted butter
⅜ cup cocoa powder
⅔ cup firmly packed brown sugar
½ teaspoon vanilla extract
¼ cup mashed plums
⅔ cup white rice flour
⅓ cup Ener-G potato flour
½ teaspoon baking soda
⅛ teaspoon sea salt
¼ cup powdered sugar

Comparative Analysis

Consider other substitutions, too. This analysis allows for all-purpose flour and plums canned in juice; powdered sugar is omitted: Calories: 58; Protein: 1g; Carbohydrates: 11g; Fat: 1g; Saturated fat: 1g; Cholesterol: 3mg; Sodium: 41mg; Fiber: 1g; PCF Ratio: 6-74-20; Exchange Approx.: 1 Carbohydrate.

1. In microwave-safe cup, combine flaxseed and water; microwave on high for 15–30 seconds. Stir the mixture. (It should have the consistency of a thick egg white; this mixture is an egg substitute.)

2. Add butter to microwave-safe mixing bowl; microwave for 15–20 seconds, until butter is melted. Add cocoa; blend into butter. Mix in flaxseed mixture, brown sugar, and vanilla.

3. Add mashed plums to other ingredients; stir to combine. (If you wish to remove plum skins, push fruit through mesh sieve. Skins add some fiber to snack, but you may not like how they look. You can use food processor to pulverize plum skins.) Blend in flours, baking soda, and salt until dough forms. Refrigerate for 1–2 hours, or until mixture is firm enough to shape into balls.

4. Preheat oven to 350°F. Form a heaping teaspoon of dough into ball; roll in powdered sugar. Place on ungreased cookie sheet; use back of fork to flatten each cookie. Bake for 8–10 minutes, or until firm. Cool completely on wire racks.

Honey Raisin Bars

PER SERVING: Calories: 71 | Protein: 1 g | Carbohydrates: 12 g | Fat: 2 g | Saturated Fat: 0 g | Cholesterol: 0 mg
Sodium: 39 mg | Fiber: 1 g | PCF Ratio: 7-66-26 | Exchange Approx.: ½ Starch, ½ Misc. Carbohydrate

INGREDIENTS | YIELDS 18 BARS; SERVING SIZE: 1 BAR

½ cup unbleached all-purpose flour
¼ teaspoon baking soda
1/8 teaspoon sea salt
¼ teaspoon cinnamon
¾ cup quick-cooking oatmeal
1 egg white, slightly beaten
2½ tablespoons sunflower oil
¼ cup honey
¼ cup skim milk
½ teaspoon vanilla
½ cup golden raisins

Tip

If you like chewier cookies or need to cut the fat in your diet, you can substitute applesauce, plums, prunes, or mashed banana for the sunflower oil.

1. Preheat oven to 350°F.

2. Sift flour, soda, salt, and cinnamon together into bowl; stir in oatmeal.

3. In another bowl, mix egg white, oil, honey, milk, vanilla, and raisins; add to liquid ingredients.

4. Drop by teaspoonful onto cookie sheets treated with nonstick spray; bake for 12–15 minutes. (Longer baking time will result in crispier cookies.) Cool on baking rack.

5. For cookie bars, spread mixture in an even layer on piece of parchment paper placed on cookie sheet; bake for 15–18 minutes. Cool slightly, then use sharp knife or pizza cutter to slice into 18 equal pieces (6 down, 3 across).

Resources

As you learn more about diabetes, you may have more questions or want to find additional information. The following resources provide a wealth of information regarding diabetes in general, as well as diets, forums, and frequently asked questions.

Recommended Websites:

ASK THE DIETITIAN
www.dietitian.com
Joanne Larsen, MS, RD, LD, maintains this site. Post specific diet-related questions or read the answers to questions from other visitors.

AMERICAN DIABETES ASSOCIATION
www.diabetes.org
This site, maintained by the recognized authority on diabetes, is dedicated to providing up-to-date information regarding medications and diabetes research findings.

AMERICAN DIETETIC ASSOCIATION
www.eatright.org
The American Dietetic Association is the world's largest organization of food and nutrition professionals. This site provides nutrition information and resources on a variety of topics and includes a tool to find a dietitian in your area.

DLIFE
www.dLife.com
An interactive diabetes website that includes diabetes information, tips for healthy eating, recipe bank, and diabetic community.

NATIONAL INSTITUTE OF DIABETES & DIGESTIVE & KIDNEY DISEASE
www.niddk.nih.gov
Site for general diabetes information, where brochures and articles can be downloaded.

THE U.S. NATIONAL LIBRARY OF MEDICINE AND NATIONAL INSTITUTE OF HEALTH
www.nlm.nih.gov/medlineplus/diabetes.html
This site has research, references, interactive tutorial, consumer materials, and guidebooks to download or order online.

CHANGING LIFE WITH DIABETES
www.changingdiabetes-us.com
An interactive website with menu-planning tools and information about different types of insulin.

Online Sources for Ingredients and Equipment

The quality of the foods you prepare is based on the quality of the ingredients you use; that's elementary. The equipment you use can make a difference, too. Even if you don't have a gourmet grocery or cooking supply store nearby, you don't have to forgo using out-of-the-ordinary ingredients or products you've been wanting to try. Chances are you can order it online through one of these sites:

Chef's Catalog
www.chefscatalog.com

McCormick Spice
www.mccormick.com

Bob's Red Mill
www.bobsredmill.com

King Arthur Flours
www.kingarthurflours.com

Cabot Cheese
www.cabotcheese.coop

Ancient Harvest
www.quinoa.net

Mrs. Dash
www.mrsdash.com

MexGrocer.com
www.mexgrocer.com

Barilla Plus Pasta
www.barillaus.com

Visit these sites to find a location near you:

Whole Foods Market
www.wholefoodsmarket.com

Trader Joe's
www.traderjoes.com

Local Harvest
www.localharvest.org
Use this website to find farmers' markets, family farms, and other sources of sustainably grown food in your area, where you can buy produce, grass-fed meats, and many other locally grown foods.

Exchange List

Because food exchange lists can be an important part of arriving at individualized meal plans, this appendix covers many of the common foods found on such lists. Please remember that the information contained in this book is not intended as medical advice. Consult your dietitian with any questions or details regarding the diet he or she has designed specifically for you. The information presented here is intended as a general guide only.

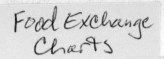
Food Exchange Charts

KEY

† = 3 grams or more of fiber per serving

‡ = High in sodium; if more than 1 serving is eaten, these foods have 400mg or more of sodium.

1 Carbohydrate Exchange List choice = 15g carbohydrate

1 Protein Exchange List choice = 7g protein

1 Milk Exchange List choice = 12g carbohydrate and 8g protein

1 Fat Exchange List choice = 5g fat

Starches and Bread

These are the foods found on the bottom tier of the food pyramid. Each exchange in this category contains about 15 grams of carbohydrates, 3 grams of protein, and a trace of fat, for a total of 80 calories. Serving sizes may vary. A general rule is that ½ cup of cooked cereal, grain, or pasta equals 1 exchange, and 1 ounce of a bread product is 1 serving. Those foods within this category that contain 3 grams or more of fiber are identified using a † symbol.

BREAD			
FOOD	**AMOUNT**	**FOOD**	**AMOUNT**
Plain roll, small	1 (1 ounce)	Tortilla, 6" across	1
Raisin, unfrosted	1 slice	White (including French, Italian)	1 slice (1 ounce)
Rye†, pumpernickel	1 slice (1 ounce)	Whole wheat	1 slice
CEREALS AND PASTA			
BRAN CEREALS†, CONCENTRATED			
100 percent bran	⅔ cup	Bran Chex	½ cup
All Bran	⅓ cup	Fiber One	⅔ cup
All-Bran with extra fiber	1 cup	Multi-Bran Chex	⅓ cup
Bran Buds	⅓ cup		
BRAN CEREALS†, FLAKED			
40 percent bran flakes	½ cup	Nutri-Grain	½ cup
Fortified Oat Flakes	⅓ cup	Bulgur, cooked	½ cup
CEREALS, MOST READY TO EAT			
unsweetened, plain	¾ cup	Puffed cereal, rice or wheat	1½ cups
Cheerios†	1 cup	Rice Krispies	⅔ cup
Cooked cereals	½ cup	Shredded wheat, biscuit	1 cup

CEREALS AND PASTA

FOOD	AMOUNT	FOOD	AMOUNT
Cornflakes	¾ cup	Shredded wheat, spoon size	½ cup
Frosted Flakes	¼ cup	Shredded Wheat and Bran†	½ cup
Grape Nuts	3 tablespoons	Special K	1 cup
Grits, cooked	½ cup	Total	¾ cup
Kix	1 cup	Wheat Chex†	½ cup
Life	½ cup	Wheaties†	⅔ cup

GRAINS

FOOD	AMOUNT	FOOD	AMOUNT
Barley, cooked	⅓ cup	Millet, dry	3 tablespoons
Buckwheat, cooked	½ cup	Oat bran, cooked	¼ cup
Bulgur, cooked	⅓ cup	Pasta, cooked	⅓ cup
Cornmeal, dry	2½ tablespoons	Quinoa, cooked	⅓ cup
Cornstarch	2 tablespoons	Rice, white or brown, cooked	⅓ cup
Couscous, cooked	⅓ cup	Rice, wild, cooked	½ cup
Flour	3 tablespoons	Wheat berries, cooked	⅔ cup
Kasha, cooked	⅓ cup	Wheat germ†	¼ cup (1 carb and 1 low-fat protein)

GRAINS

FOOD	AMOUNT	FOOD	AMOUNT
Barley, cooked	⅓ cup	Millet, dry	3 tablespoons
Buckwheat, cooked	½ cup	Oat bran, cooked	¼ cup
Bulgur, cooked	⅓ cup	Pasta, cooked	⅓ cup
Cornmeal, dry	2½ tablespoons	Quinoa, cooked	⅓ cup
Cornstarch	2 tablespoons	Rice, white or brown, cooked	⅓ cup
Couscous, cooked	⅓ cup	Rice, wild, cooked	½ cup
Flour	3 tablespoons	Wheat berries, cooked	⅔ cup
Kasha, cooked	⅓ cup	Wheat germ†	¼ cup (1 carb and 1 low-fat protein)

CRACKERS AND SNACKS

FOOD	AMOUNT	FOOD	AMOUNT
Club, reduced fat	6	Pretzels‡	¾ ounce
Graham crackers, (2½" square)	3	Rye crisp, 2" × 3½"	4
Matzoh	1 (¾ ounce)	Saltine-type crackers‡	6
Matzoh with bran	1 (¾ ounce)	Snack-Well's, fat-free, cheddar‡	24
Manischewitz whole-wheat matzoh crackers	7	Snack-Well's, fat-free, cracked pepper	8
Melba toast, rectangles	5	Snack-Well's, fat-free, wheat	6

CRACKERS AND SNACKS *continued*

Food	Amount	Food	Amount
Melba toast, rounds	10	Wasa Hearty Rye	2
Orville Redenbacher Smart Pop! popcorn	3 cups	Wasa Lite	2
Popcorn, air popped, no fat added	3 cups	Wasa Golden Rye	2
Town House, reduced fat‡	8		

DRIED BEANS, LENTILS, AND PEAS *Note: All portions given are for cooked amounts.*

FOOD	AMOUNT	FOOD	AMOUNT
Baked beans†	⅓ cup	Lima beans†	⅔ cup
Beans†, white	½ cup	Navy beans†	½ cup
Chickpeas/Garbanzo beans†	½ cup	Peas†, black-eyed	½ cup
Kidney beans†	½ cup	Peas†, split	½ cup
Lentils†	½ cup	Pinto beans†	½ cup

STARCHY VEGETABLES

FOOD	AMOUNT	FOOD	AMOUNT
Corn†	½ cup	Potato, baked or boiled	1 small (3 ounce)
Corn on the cob†, 6" long	1	Potato, mashed	½ cup
Lima beans†	½ cup	Pumpkin	1 cup
Mixed vegetables, with corn or peas	⅔ cup	Squash, winter (acorn, butternut)	1 cup
Peas†, green (canned or frozen)	½ cup	Yam, sweet potato	½ cup
Plantain†	½ cup		

STARCHES AND BREADS PREPARED WITH FAT *These count as 1 starch/bread plus 1 fat choice*

FOOD	AMOUNT	FOOD	AMOUNT
Biscuit, 2½" across	1	Pancake, 4" across	2
Chow mein noodles	½ cup	Stuffing, bread (prepared)	¼ cup
Corn bread, 2" cube	1 (2 ounce)	Taco shell, 6" across	2
French fries (2" to 3" long)	10 (1½ ounces)	Waffle, 4½" square	1
Muffin, plain, small	1		

CRACKERS

FOOD	AMOUNT	FOOD	AMOUNT
Arrowroot	4	Ritz‡	7
Butter cracker‡, round	7	Sociables‡	9
Butter cracker‡, rectangle	6	Stella D'oro Sesame Breadsticks	2
Cheese Nips‡	20	Sunshine HiHo‡	6
Cheez-It‡	27	Teddy Grahams	15
Club‡	6	Tidbits‡	21
Combos‡	1 ounce	Triscuits‡	5
Escort‡	5	Town House‡	6
Lorna Doone	3	Vanilla Wafers	6
Meal Mates‡	5	Wasa Breakfast crispbread	2

CRACKERS *continued*			
Oyster‡	20	Wasa Fiber Plus crispbread	4
Peanut butter crackers‡	3	Wasa Sesame crispbread	2
Pepperidge Farm Bordeaux cookies	3	Waverly Wafers‡	2
Pepperidge Farm Goldfish‡	36	Wheat Thins, reduced fat‡	13
Popcorn, microwave, light	4 cups		

Vegetables

Vegetables fall within the second tier of the food pyramid. Each vegetable serving is calculated to contain 5 grams of carbohydrates, 2 grams of protein, between 2 to 3 grams of fiber, and 25 calories. Vegetables are a good source of vitamins and minerals. Fresh or frozen vegetables are preferred because of their higher vitamin and mineral content; however, canned vegetables are also acceptable, with the preference being for low-sodium or salt-free varieties. As a general rule, one Vegetable Exchange is usually equal to ½ cup cooked, 1 cup raw, or ½ cup juice. Not all vegetables are found on the Vegetable Exchange List. Starchy vegetables such as corn, peas, and potatoes are part of the Starches and Bread Exchange List. Vegetables with fewer than 10 calories per serving are found on the Free Food Exchange List.

VEGETABLE EXCHANGE LIST *Cooked or steamed serving.*					
FOOD	**AMOUNT**	**FOOD**	**AMOUNT**	**FOOD**	**AMOUNT**
Bean sprouts	½ cup	Kohlrabi	½ cup	Tomato	1 medium
Beet greens	½ cup	Leeks	½ cup	Tomato, canned‡	½ cup
Beets	½ cup	Mushrooms, fresh	1 cup	Tomato, paste‡	1½ tablespoons
Broccoli	½ cup	Mustard greens	1 cup	Tomato sauce, canned‡	⅓ cup
Brussels sprouts	½ cup	Okra	½ cup	Tomato/vegetable juice‡	½ cup
Cabbage	1 cup	Onions	½ cup	Turnip greens	1 cup
Carrots	½ cup	Pea pods	½ cup	Turnips	½ cup
Cauliflower	½ cup	Radishes	1 cup	Tomato/vegetable juice‡	½ cup
Celery	1 cup	Red pepper	1 cup	Turnip greens	1 cup
Collard greens	1 cup	Rutabaga	½ cup	Turnips	½ cup
Eggplant	½ cup	Sauerkraut‡	½ cup	Water chestnuts	6 whole or ½ cup
Fennel leaf	1 cup	Spaghetti sauce, jar	¼ cup	Wax beans	½ cup
Green beans	1 cup	Spaghetti squash	½ cup	Zucchini	1 cup
Green pepper	1 cup	Spinach	½ cup		
Kale	½ cup	Summer squash	1 cup		

Fruits

One Fruit Exchange has about 15 grams of carbohydrates, which totals 60 calories. The serving sizes for fruits vary considerably, so consult the list. Also, note that portion amounts are given for fruit that is dried, fresh, frozen, or canned packed in its own juice with no sugar added.

FRESH, FROZEN, AND UNSWEETENED CANNED FRUIT

FOOD	AMOUNT	FOOD	AMOUNT
Apple, raw, 2" across	1	Guavas, small	1½
Apple, dried	4 rings	Honeydew melon, medium	⅛
Applesauce, unsweetened	½ cup	Honeydew melon, cubes	1 cup
Apricots, canned	4 halves or ½ cup	Kiwi, large	1
Apricots, dried	8 halves	Kumquats, medium	5
Apricots, fresh, medium	4	Loquats, fresh	12
Banana, 9" long	½	Lychees, dried or fresh	10
Banana flakes or chips	3 tablespoons	Mandarin oranges	¾ cup
Blackberries, raw	¾ cup	Mango, small	½
Blueberries†, raw	¾ cup	Nectarine, 2½" across	1
Boysenberries	1 cup	Orange, 3" across	1
Canned fruit, unless otherwise stated	½ cup	Papaya, fresh, 3½" across	½
Cantaloupe, 5" across	⅓	Papaya, fresh, cubed	1 cup
Cantaloupe, cubes	1 cup	Peach, 2¾" across	1 peach or ¾ cup
Casaba, 7" across	⅙ melon	Peaches, canned	2 halves or 1 cup
Casaba, cubed	1⅓ cups	Pears, canned	2 halves or ½ cup
Cherries, large, raw	12 whole	Persimmon, medium, native	2
Cherries, canned	½ cup	Pineapple, raw	¾ cup
Cherries, dried (no sugar added)	2 tablespoons	Pineapple, canned	⅓ cup
Cranberries, dried (no sugar added)	2 tablespoons	Plantain, cooked	⅓ cup
Currants	2 tablespoons	Pomegranate†	½
Dates	3	Prunes, dried, medium	3
Fig, dried	1	Raisins	2 tablespoons
Figs, fresh, 2" across	2	Plum, raw, 2" across	2
Fruit cocktail, canned	½ cup	Raspberries†, raw	1 cup
Grapefruit, medium	½	Strawberries†, raw, whole	1¼ cups
Grapefruit, sections	¾ cup	Tangerine, 2½" across	2
Grapes, small	15	Watermelon, cubes	1¼ cups

DRIED FRUIT†			
†Apples	4 rings	†Figs	1½
†Apricots	8 halves	†Prunes, medium	3
Dates, medium	2½	Raisins	2 tablespoons
FRUIT JUICE			
Apple cider	½ cup	Grapefruit juice	½ cup
Apple juice, unsweetened	½ cup	Grape juice	⅓ cup
Cranapple juice, unsweetened	⅜ cup	Orange juice	½ cup
Cranberry juice cocktail	⅓ cup	Pineapple juice	½ cup
Cranberry juice, low-calorie	1⅛ cups	Prune juice	⅓ cup
Cranberry juice, unsweetened	½ cup		

Milk

Milk servings are usually marked at 1 cup or 8 ounces. Like meats, Milk Exchange Lists are divided into categories depending on the fat content of the choices. Each Milk Exchange has about 12 grams of carbohydrate and 8 grams of protein; however, the calories in each exchange will vary according to the fat content.

SKIM OR VERY LOW-FAT MILK			
FOOD	**AMOUNT**	**FOOD**	**AMOUNT**
½% milk	1 cup	Skim milk	1 cup
1% milk	1 cup	Skim milk, evaporated	½ cup
Buttermilk, low-fat or 1%	1 cup	Yogurt, plain, nonfat	8 ounces
Nonfat milk, dry	⅓ cup		
LOW-FAT MILK			
2% milk	1 cup	Yogurt, plain, low-fat with added nonfat milk solids	8 ounces
WHOLE MILK			
Whole milk	1 cup	Yogurt, plain, whole milk	8 ounces
Whole milk, evaporated	½ cup		

The whole-milk group has much more fat per serving than the skim and low-fat groups. Whole milk has more than 3¼ percent butterfat, so you should limit your choices from this group as much as possible.

Meats

Each serving of meat or meat substitute has about 7 grams of protein. As shown in the tables below, the Meats Exchange Lists are divided depending on the fat content of the meat or meat substitute choice. (See Chapter 5 for suggestions on the healthiest ways to prepare meats.)

Make your selections from the lean and medium-fat meat, poultry, and fish choices in your meal plan as much as possible. This helps you keep the fat intake in your diet low, which may help decrease your risk for heart disease. Remember that the meats in the high-fat group have more saturated fat, cholesterol, and calories, so you should consult with your dietitian about whether or not your diet should include any meats from that group. When they are permitted, most dietitians recommend limiting your choices from the high-fat group to a maximum of three times per week.

Meats and meat substitutes that have 400 milligrams or more of sodium per exchange are indicated with the ‡ symbol.

Meats Exchange List portions are generally 1 ounce of cooked meat (using the 4 ounces of raw meat results in 3 ounces of cooked meat standard). Beef, pork, fish, poultry, cheese, eggs, and, when they're used as meat substitutes, dried beans, legumes, and some nuts, fall within the Meats Exchange Lists categories. Because the calorie counts vary so widely (as does the cholesterol and saturated fat content), your dietitian will advise from which lists you are to choose your selections.

EXCHANGE	CARBOHYDRATE	PROTEIN (G)	FAT(G)	CALORIES
Very-Lean Meats	0	7	0–1	35
Lean Meats	0	7	3	55
Medium-Fat	0	7	5	75
High-Fat	0	7	8	100

VERY-LEAN MEATS (AND MEAT SUBSTITUTES)

Meats in this category are usually the reduced-fat varieties, like Healthy Choice, and contain 4 percent or fewer calories from fat, which unless otherwise noted below are at 1 ounce per Food Exchange List portion. Name-brand foods come and go, with new ones introduced regularly that phase out others. Check product labels or ask your dietitian to ascertain which products currently fall within this category. One choice provides about 35–45 calories, 7 grams of protein, no carbohydrates, and 0–2 grams of fat.

FOOD	AMOUNT	FOOD	AMOUNT
Buffalo	1 ounce	Fish and seafood, fresh or frozen, cooked: clams, cod, crab, flounder, haddock, halibut, imitation crabmeat, lobster, scallops, shrimp, trout, tuna (in water)	2 ounces
Chicken, white meat, skinless	1 ounce	Ostrich	1 ounce

VERY-LEAN MEATS (AND MEAT SUBSTITUTES) *continued*

FOOD	AMOUNT	FOOD	AMOUNT
Cornish hen, white meat, skinless	1 ounce	Turkey, ground, 93–99 percent fat free	1 ounce
Cottage cheese, fat free or 1%	¼ cup	Turkey, white meat, skinless	1 ounce
Ricotta, 100 percent fat free‡	1 ounce	Turkey sausage, 97 percent fat free‡	1 ounce
Egg substitute, plain (if less than 40 calories per serving)	¼ cup	Venison	1 ounce

LEAN MEATS (AND MEAT SUBSTITUTES) *One choice provides about 55 calories, 7 grams of protein, no carbohydrates, and 3 grams of fat.*

FOOD	AMOUNT	FOOD	AMOUNT
95 percent fat-free luncheon meat	1 ounce		
BEEF, OF LEAN BEEF SUCH AS:			
Chipped beef‡ (USDA Good or Choice grade)	1 ounce	Pheasant, without skin	1 ounce
Flank steak (USDA Good or Choice grade)	1 ounce	Boiled ham‡	1 ounce
Round steak (USDA Good or Choice grade)	1 ounce	Canadian bacon‡	1 ounce
Sirloin steak (USDA Good or Choice grade)	1 ounce	Canned ham‡	1 ounce
Tenderloin (USDA Good or Choice grade)	1 ounce	Cured ham‡	1 ounce
Clams, fresh or canned in water‡	2 ounces	Fresh ham	1 ounce
Cottage cheese, any variety	¼ cup	Tenderloin	1 ounce
Crab	2 ounces	Chicken, dark meat, without skin	1 ounce
Diet cheese‡ (with fewer than 55 calories per ounce)	1 ounce	Cornish game hen, dark meat, without skin	1 ounce
Duck, without skin	1 ounce	Turkey, dark meat, without skin	1 ounce
Egg substitutes (with fewer than 55 calories per ¼ cup)	¼ cup	Rabbit	1 ounce
Egg whites	3	Sardines, canned, medium	2
Fish, all fresh and frozen catfish, salmon, and other fattier fish	1 ounce	Scallops	2 ounces
Goose, without skin	1 ounce	Shrimp	2 ounces
Grated Parmesan	2 tablespoons	Squirrel	1 ounce
Herring, uncreamed or smoked	1 ounce	Tofu	3 ounces
Lobster	2 ounces	Veal, all cuts are lean except for veal cutlets (ground or cubed)	1 ounce
Oysters, medium	6	Venison	1 ounce

MEDIUM-FAT MEATS (AND MEAT SUBSTITUTES) One choice provides about 75 calories, 7 grams of protein, no carbohydrates, and 5 grams of fat.

FOOD	AMOUNT	FOOD	AMOUNT
86 percent fat-free luncheon meat‡	1 ounce	Lamb chops	1 ounce
Chuck roast	1 ounce	Lamb leg	1 ounce
Cubed steak	1 ounce	Lamb roast	1 ounce
Ground beef	1 ounce	Liver (high in cholesterol)	1 ounce
Meat loaf	1 ounce	Parmesan cheese‡	3 tablespoons
Porterhouse steak	1 ounce	Pork chops	1 ounce
Rib roast	1 ounce	Pork loin roast	1 ounce
Rump roast	1 ounce	Boston butt	1 ounce
T-bone steak	1 ounce	Pork cutlets	1 ounce
Diet cheeses‡ (with 56–80 calories per ounce)	1 ounce	Chicken (with skin)	1 ounce
Mozzarella (skim or part-skim milk)	1 ounce	Duck, domestic, well drained of fat	1 ounce
Ricotta (skim or part-skim milk)	¼ cup	Goose, domestic, well drained of fat	1 ounce
Egg (high in cholesterol, so limit to 3 per week)	1	Ground turkey	1 ounce
Egg substitutes (with 56–80 calories per ¼ cup)	¼ cup	Romano cheese	3 tablespoons
Heart (high in cholesterol)	1 ounce	Sweetbreads (high in cholesterol)	1 ounce
Kidney (high in cholesterol)	1 ounce	Salmon‡, canned	¼ cup
Lamb chops	1 ounce	Tofu (2½" × 2¾" × 1")	4 ounce
Lamb leg	1 ounce	Tuna‡, canned in oil, drained	¼ cup
Lamb roast	1 ounce	Veal cutlet, ground or cubed, unbreaded	1 ounce

Remember, these items are high in saturated fat, cholesterol, and calories, and should be eaten only three or fewer times per week. One choice provides about 100 calories, 7 grams of protein, no carbohydrates, and 8 grams of fat. One exchange choice is equal to any one of the following items:

HIGH-FAT MEATS (AND MEAT SUBSTITUTES)		CHEESE, ALL REGULAR CHEESE‡	
FOOD	AMOUNT	FOOD	AMOUNT
Most USDA Prime cuts of beef	1 ounce	American	1 ounce
Beef‡, corned	1 ounce	Bleu	1 ounce
Ribs, beef	1 ounce	Cheddar	1 ounce
Bologna‡	1 ounce	Monterey	1 ounce
		Swiss	1 ounce

FOOD	AMOUNT	FOOD	AMOUNT
Chicken hot dog, 10/pound	1 frank	Lamb, ground	1 ounce
Turkey hot dog, 10/pound	1 frank	Peanut butter (contains unsaturated fat)	1 tablespoon

FOOD	AMOUNT	FOOD	AMOUNT
Pimiento loaf‡	1 ounce	Spareribs	1 ounce
Pork chop	1 ounce	Steak	1 ounce
Pork, ground	1 ounce	Salami‡	1 ounce

SAUSAGE‡			
Bratwurst‡	1 ounce	Polish	1 ounce
Italian	1 ounce	Pork sausage‡ (patty or link)	1 ounce
Knockwurst, smoked	1 ounce		

Counts as one high-fat meat plus one fat exchange:	
Hot dog‡—beef, pork, or combination, 400mg or more of sodium per exchange, 10/pound	1 frank

Fats

Each Fats Exchange List serving will contain about 5 grams of fat and 45 calories. Fats are found in margarine, butter, oils, nuts, meat fat, and dairy products. Saturated fat amounts and sodium contents can vary considerably, depending on the choice. Most dietitians recommend polyunsaturated or monounsaturated fats whenever possible.

UNSATURATED FATS			
FOOD	AMOUNT	FOOD	AMOUNT
Almonds, dry roasted	6	Pine nuts	1 tablespoon
Avocado, medium	⅛	Peanuts, small	20
Cashews, dry roasted	1 tablespoon or 6	Pecan halves	4
Cooking oil (corn, cottonseed, safflower, soybean, sunflower, olive, peanut)	1 teaspoon	Pistachio	12
Hazelnuts (filberts)	5	Pumpkin seeds	2 teaspoons
Macadamia nuts	3	Salad dressing, all varieties, regular	1 tablespoon
Margarine	1 teaspoon	Salad dressing, mayonnaise-type, reduced calorie	1 tablespoon
Margarine, diet‡	1 tablespoon	Salad dressing, mayonnaise-type, regular	2 teaspoons
Mayonnaise	1 teaspoon	Salad dressing, reduced calorie‡ (2 tablespoons of low-calorie dressing is a free food)	2 tablespoons
Mayonnaise, reduced calorie‡	1 tablespoon	Sesame seeds	1 tablespoon
Olives, black, large‡	9	Sunflower seeds, without shells	1 tablespoon

UNSATURATED FATS continued

FOOD	AMOUNT	FOOD	AMOUNT
Olives, green, large‡	10	Tahini	2 teaspoons
Other nuts	1 tablespoon	Walnut halves	4
Peanuts, large	10		

SATURATED FATS

FOOD	AMOUNT	FOOD	AMOUNT
Bacon‡	1 slice	Cream, heavy	1 tablespoon
Butter	1 teaspoon	Cream, light, coffee, table	2 tablespoons
Butter, whipped	2 teaspoons	Cream, sour	2 tablespoons
Chitterlings	½ ounce	Cream, whipping	1 tablespoon
Coconut, shredded	2 tablespoons	Cream cheese	1 tablespoon
Coffee whitener, liquid	2 tablespoons	Salt pork‡	¼ ounce
Coffee whitener, powder	4 tablespoons		

Free Foods

A free food is any food or drink that contains less than 20 calories per serving. Unless a serving size is specified, you can eat as much as you want of these foods. You are limited to eating two or three servings per day of those foods with a specific serving size.

FREE DRINKS

FOOD	AMOUNT	FOOD	AMOUNT
Bouillon or canned broth without fat‡		Cocoa powder, unsweetened	1 tablespoon
Bouillon, low sodium		Coffee	
Broth, low sodium		Drink mixes, sugar free	
Carbonated drinks, sugar free		Tea	
Carbonated water		Tonic water, sugar free	
Club soda			

FREE FRUITS AND VEGETABLES

FOOD	AMOUNT	FOOD	AMOUNT
Cranberries, unsweetened	½ cup	Green onion	
Rhubarb, unsweetened	½ cup	Hot peppers	
Vegetables, raw	1 cup	Lettuce	
Alfalfa sprouts		Mushrooms	
Cabbage		Parsley	
Celery		Pickles, unsweetened‡	
Chinese cabbage†		Pimiento	

FREE FRUITS AND VEGETABLES *continued*			
Cucumber		Romaine	
Endive		Salad greens	
Escarole		Zucchini†	
Radishes		Watercress	
Spinach			

FREE SWEETS			
FOOD	**AMOUNT**	**FOOD**	**AMOUNT**
Candy, hard, sugar free		Jam/jelly, sugar free	2 teaspoons
Gelatin, sugar free		Pancake syrup, sugar free	1–2 tablespoons
Gum, sugar free		Sugar substitutes (saccharin, aspartame, Splenda)	
Jam/jelly, low sugar	2 teaspoons	Whipped topping	2 tablespoons

FREE CONDIMENTS			
FOOD	**AMOUNT**	**FOOD**	**AMOUNT**
Horseradish		Pickles, dill, unsweetened‡	
Ketchup	1 tablespoon	Salad dressing, low calorie	2 tablespoons
Mustard		Taco sauce	1 tablespoon
Nonstick pan spray		Vinegar	

FREE SEASONINGS		
FOOD		
Basil	Lime	Pepper
Celery seeds	Hot pepper sauce	Pimiento
Chili powder	Lemon	Soy sauce, low sodium ("lite")
Chives	Lemon juice	Soy sauce‡
Cinnamon	Lemon pepper	Spices
Curry	Lime juice	Wine, used in cooking amount ¼ cup
Dill	Mint	Worcestershire sauce‡
Garlic	Onion powder	
Garlic powder	Oregano	
Herbs	Paprika	
FREE FLAVORING EXTRACTS		
Almond	Peppermint	Lemon
Butter	Vanilla	Walnut

Seasonings can be very helpful in making foods taste better, but be careful how much sodium you use. Read labels to help you choose seasonings that do not contain sodium or salt.

MEAT SUBSTITUTE PROTEIN FOODS Note: Foods on this list equal 1 Protein Food Exchange List serving (0g carb, 7g protein, 0–5 gfat).	
FOOD	AMOUNT
Egg substitute	¼ cup
Soy cheese	1 ounce
Tofu, firm	½ cup (4 ounces)

BEANS USED AS A MEAT SUBSTITUTE		
FOOD	AMOUNT	EXCHANGES
Dried beans†	1 cup, cooked	1 lean meat, 2 starches
Dried lentils†	1 cup, cooked	1 lean meat, 2 starches
Dried peas†	1 cup, cooked	1 lean meat, 2 starches

NUTS AND SEEDS USED AS A MEAT SUBSTITUTE Note: Foods on this list equal 1 Protein and 2 or 3 Fat Food Exchange List serving (0g carb, 7g protein, 10–15g fat). Consult product label to determine fat content for your choice.	
Almonds	¼ cup
Pecans	¼ cup
Peanuts	¼ cup
Pine nuts	2 tablespoons
Pistachios	¼ cup (1 ounce)
Pumpkin seeds	¼ cup
Sesame seeds	¼ cup
Squash seeds	¼ cup
Sunflower seeds	¼ cup
Walnut halves	16–20

FAT FOODS USED AS A MEAT SUBSTITUTE Note: Foods on this list equal 1 Fat Food Exchange List serving (0g carb, 5g fat).		
FOOD	AMOUNT	EXCHANGES
Almond butter	1 tablespoon	2 fats
Cashew butter	1 tablespoon	2 fats
Flax seed oil	1 teaspoon	1 fat
Peanut oil	1 teaspoon	1 fat
Sesame butter	1 tablespoon	2 fats

Combination Foods

Food is often mixed together in various combinations that do not fit into only one exchange list. Each of the recipes in this book gives the exchange list exchanges for that dish. The following is included as a list of average exchange list values for some typical combination foods. Ask your dietitian for information about these or any other combination of foods you'd like to eat.

Foods for Special Treats

These foods, despite their sugar or fat content, are intended to be added to your meal plan in moderate amounts, as long as your dietitian agrees and if, despite consuming them, you can still maintain blood-glucose control. Your dietitian can also advise how often you can eat these foods. Because these special treats are concentrated sources of carbohydrate, the portion sizes are very small.

FOODS FOR SPECIAL TREATS

FOOD	AMOUNT	EXCHANGES
Angel-food cake	1/12 cake	2 starches
Cake, no icing	1/12 cake (3" square)	2 starches, 2 fats
Cookies	2 small (1¾" across)	2 starches, 1 fat
Frozen fruit yogurt	⅓ cup	1 starch
Gingersnaps	3	1 starch
Granola	¼ cup	1 starch, 1 fat
Granola bars	1 small	1 starch, 1 fat
Ice cream, any flavor	½ cup	1 starch, 2 fats
Ice milk, any flavor	½ cup	1 starch, 1 fat
Sherbet, any flavor	¼ cup	1 starch
Snack chips‡, all varieties	1 ounce	1 starch, 2 fats
Vanilla wafers	6 small	1 starch, 2 fats

COMBO FOODS

FOOD	AMOUNT	EXCHANGES
Bean soup†‡	1 cup (8 ounces)	1 lean meat, 1 starch, 1 vegetable
Casserole,	2 medium-fat meats	
Homemade casserole	1 cup (8 ounces)	2 starches, 1 fat
Cheese pizza‡, thin crust	¼ of 15-ounce pizza	1 medium-fat meat
Cheese pizza‡, 10" pizza	2 starches, 1 fat	
Chili with beans, commercial†‡	1 cup (8 ounces)	2 medium-fat meats, 2 starches, 2 fats
Chow mein†‡ (without noodles or rice)	2 cups (16 ounces)	2 lean meats, 1 starch, 2 vegetables
Chunky soup, all varieties‡	10¾-ounce can	1 medium-fat meat, 1 starch, 1 vegetable
Cream soup‡ (made with water)	1 cup (8 ounces)	1 starch, 1 fat
Macaroni and cheese‡	1 cup (8 ounces)	1 medium-fat meat, 2 starches, 2 fats
Spaghetti and meatballs, canned‡	1 cup (8 ounces)	1 medium-fat meat, 1 fat, 2 starches
Sugar-free pudding (made with skim milk)	½ cup	1 starch
Vegetable soup‡	1 cup (8 ounces)	1 starch

MISCELLANEOUS FOODS				
FOOD	AMOUNT	FOOD GROUP	CARBOHYDRATE GRAMS	CALORIES
Jam, regular	1 tablespoon	1 carbohydrate	13g	80
Jelly, regular	1 tablespoon	1 carbohydrate	13g	80
Honey, regular	1 tablespoon	1 carbohydrate	13g	80
Sugar	1 tablespoon	1 carbohydrate	12g	46
Syrup, light	2 tablespoons	1 carbohydrates	13g	80
Syrup, regular	2 tablespoons	2 carbohydrates	27g	160
Yogurt, regular, with fruit	1 cup	3 carbohydrates	45g	240

OTHER SPECIAL FOODS		
FOOD	AMOUNT	EXCHANGES
Brewer's yeast	3 tablespoons	1 bread
Carob flour	⅛ cup	1 bread
Kefir	1 cup	1 milk, 1 fat
Miso	3 tablespoons	1 bread, ½ lean meat
Sea vegetables, cooked	½ cup	1 vegetable
Soy flour	¼ cup	1 lean meat, ½ bread
Soy grits, raw	⅛ cup	1 lean meat
Soy milk	1 cup	1 milk, 1 fat
Tahini	1 teaspoon	1 fat
Tempeh	4 ounces	1 bread, 2 protein
Wheat germ	1 tablespoon	½ bread

Measuring Foods

Portion control is an important part of implementing a diet based on the Food Exchange Lists. This helps ensure you eat the right serving sizes of food. Liquids and some solid foods (such as tuna, cottage cheese, and canned fruits) can be measured using a measuring cup. Measuring spoons are useful to guarantee correct amounts for foods used in smaller portions, like oil, salad dressing, and peanut butter. A scale can be very useful for measuring almost anything, especially meat, poultry, and fish.

Similar in manner to how professional chefs cook, you will eventually learn how to estimate food amounts. Until then, it can be useful to remember that 1 cup is about equal in size to an average woman's closed fist. A thumb is about the size of 1 table-spoon or a 1-ounce portion of cheese. The tip of the thumb equals about 1 teaspoon, a useful gauge when trying to determine how much butter to add to your bread or dressing to add to a salad when you're dining out and don't have measuring spoons available.

Many raw foods will weigh less after they are cooked. This is especially true for most meats. On the other hand, starches often swell during cooking, so a small amount of uncooked starch results in a much larger amount of cooked food. Some examples of those changes are:

STARCH GROUP	UNCOOKED	COOKED
Cream of wheat	2 level tablespoons	½ cup
Dried beans	3 tablespoons	⅓ cup
Dried peas	3 tablespoons	⅓ cup
Grits	3 level tablespoons	½ cup
Lentils	2 tablespoons	⅓ cup
Macaroni	¼ cup	½ cup
Noodles	⅓ cup	½ cup
Oatmeal	3 level tablespoons	½ cup
Rice	2 level tablespoons	⅓ cup
Spaghetti	¼ cup	½ cup
MEAT GROUP	UNCOOKED	COOKED
Chicken	1 small drumstick	1 ounce
Chicken	½ chicken breast	3 ounces
Hamburger	4 ounces	3 ounces

APPENDIX C

Herbal and Other Seasoning Mixtures

Using herbs is a delicious way to season dishes and cut the amount of salt needed for flavor, too. Although fresh herbs need to be used immediately; dried herb mixtures can be prepared in advance and stored in an airtight container. The easiest way to dry fresh herbs is to put the baking sheet in an oven at 200°F–225°F for 1 hour. Blends made from whole seeds or leaves usually need to be coarsely ground in a spice grinder or small food processor prior to using.

Barbecue Blend

4 tablespoons dried basil
4 tablespoons dried rubbed sage
4 tablespoons dried thyme
4 teaspoons cracked black pepper
4 teaspoons dried savory
1 teaspoon dried lemon peel

Cajun Blend

2 tablespoons paprika
1½ tablespoons garlic powder
1 tablespoon onion powder
½ tablespoon black pepper
2 teaspoons cayenne pepper
2 teaspoons dried oregano
2 teaspoons dried thyme

Cabbean Blend

1 tablespoon curry powder
1 tablespoon ground cumin
1 tablespoon ground allspice
1 tablespoon ground ginger
1 teaspoon ground cayenne pepper

Country Blend

5 teaspoons dried thyme
4 teaspoons dried basil
4 teaspoons dried chervil
4 teaspoons dried tarragon

Fish and Seafood Herbs

5 teaspoons dried basil
5 teaspoons crushed fennel seed
4 teaspoons dried parsley
1 teaspoon dried lemon peel

French Blend

1 tablespoon crushed dried tarragon
1 tablespoon crushed dried chervil
1 tablespoon onion powder

Herbes de Provence

4 teaspoons dried oregano
2 teaspoons dried basil
2 teaspoons dried sweet marjoram
2 teaspoons dried thyme
1 teaspoon dried mint
1 teaspoon dried rosemary
1 teaspoon dried sage leaves
1 teaspoon fennel seed
1 teaspoon dried lavender (optional)

Italian Blend

1 tablespoon crushed dried basil
1 tablespoon crushed dried thyme
1 tablespoon crushed dried oregano
2 tablespoons garlic powder

Mediterranean Blend

1 tablespoon dried sun-ded tomatoes
1 tablespoon dried basil
1 teaspoon dried oregano
1 teaspoon dried thyme
1 tablespoon garlic powder

TIP: If you don't have a food processor, you can freeze the sun-dried tomatoes so they will be easier to crush; however, that adds moisture to the herb blend, so it can't be stored.

Middle Eastern Blend

1 tablespoon ground coriander
1 tablespoon ground cumin
1 tablespoon turmec
1 teaspoon ground cinnamon
1 teaspoon crushed dried mint

Old Bay Seasoning

1 tablespoon celery seed
1 tablespoon whole black peppercorns
6 bay leaves
½ teaspoon whole cardamom
½ teaspoon mustard seed
4 whole cloves
1 teaspoon sweet Hungaan paprika
¼ teaspoon mace

Pacific Rim

1 tablespoon Chinese five-spice powder
1 tablespoon paprika
1 tablespoon ground ginger
1 teaspoon black pepper

Sonoran Blend

1 tablespoon ground chili powder
1 tablespoon black pepper
1 tablespoon crushed dried oregano
1 tablespoon crushed dried thyme
1 tablespoon crushed dried coander
1 tablespoon garlic powder

Stuffing Blend

6 tablespoons dried rubbed sage
3 tablespoons dried sweet marjoram
2 tablespoons dried parsley
4 teaspoons dried celery flakes

Texas Seasoning

3 tablespoons dried cilantro
2 tablespoons dried oregano
4 teaspoons dried thyme
2 tablespoons pure good-quality chili powder
2 tablespoons freshly ground black pepper
2 tablespoons ground cumin
2 small crushed dried chili peppers
1 teaspoon garlic powder

Index

We Have
EVERYTHING®
on Anything!

With more than 19 million copies sold, the Everything® series has become one of America's favorite resources for solving problems, learning new skills, and organizing lives. Our brand is not only recognizable—it's also welcomed.

The series is a hand-in-hand partner for people who are ready to tackle new subjects—like you!

For more information on the Everything® series, please visit *www.adamsmedia.com*.

The Everything® list spans a wide range of subjects, with more than 500 titles covering 25 different categories:

Business	History	Reference
Careers	Home Improvement	Religion
Children's Storybooks	Everything Kids	Self-Help
Computers	Languages	Sports & Fitness
Cooking	Music	Travel
Crafts and Hobbies	New Age	Wedding
Education/Schools	Parenting	Writing
Games and Puzzles	Personal Finance	
Health	Pets	